"*Gayle is one of America's top nutritionists. Her program teaches you how small changes can help you achieve your goals—it is inspirational.*"

DEAN ORNISH, M.D.
Founder and President, Preventive Medicine Research Institute
Clinical Professor of Medicine, University of California, San Francisco
Author, *Dr. Dean Ornish's Program for Reversing Heart Disease* and *Eat More, Weigh Less*

"*An outstanding presentation of how improved nutrition and eating habits can enhance overall health and well-being.*"

CHARLES D. GERSON, M.D.
Gastroenterologist, The Mind-Body Digestive Center
Associate Clinical Professor of Medicine, Mt. Sinai School of Medicine

"*Gayle's approach is based on the fact that how we live on a day-to-day basis has an enormous impact on our health, well-being, and happiness. Active Wellness teaches you how to create a personally satisfying daily routine enabling you to reach your goals to lose weight, stay well, and prevent illness.*"

ELSA-GRACE V. GIARDINA, M.D.
Medical Director, Center for Women's Health
Professor of Clinical Medicine/Cardiology, Columbia Presbyterian Medical Center

"*Gayle Reichler's Active Wellness Program provides both a philosophy of life and a pragmatic guide to the type of healthy lifestyle that makes preventing cardiovascular disease and obesity enjoyable, rewarding, and fun. Reducing obesity reduces high blood pressure, blood sugar, cholesterol, triglycerides, risk of colon and breast cancer, and addresses the two major epidemics of obesity and diabetes that Americans face in the first decade of the twenty-first century.*"

BRADLEY A. RADWANER, M.D., FACC
Director, The New York Center for the Prevention of Heart Disease

"As a top wellness coach and leading nutritionist, Gayle Reichler's expertise and guidance have been invaluable. Gayle has been instrumental in rolling out Avon's wellness initiative and in communicating Avon's message of a healthy lifestyle through our international campaign for wellness and weight management. We are proud to work with Gayle as our wellness coach and nutritionist at her Active Wellness Center at the Avon Salon and Spa."

ANDREA JUNG
CEO and Chairman, Avon

"An inspiring and carefully planned approach to improving your health. I recommend Active Wellness to persons looking for a well-planned, attainable program."

DR. MICHELLE WARREN
Medical Director, Center for Menopause & Hormonal Disorders
Professor of Medicine and Obstetrics and Gynecology
Sloan Hospital for Women, Columbia Presbyterian Medical Center

"Gayle Reichler's Active Wellness *will guide each reader through their own personal journey, not only toward a healthy weight, but a truly holistic, healthy lifestyle. Nothing is left out, from making the best food choices to an effective approach to stress management to appropriate exercise recommendations. Ms. Reichler is a phenomenal nutritionist."*

LISA POWELL, R.D.
Nutrition Director, Canyon Ranch Spa

"Active Wellness is a comprehensive book that is outstanding for anyone desiring lifestyle changes, including people with diabetes. Gayle Reichler approaches health through the mind, body, and spirit while her recipes make it fun to be healthy."

CAROL GUBER, M.S.
Author, *Carol Guber's Type 2 Diabetes Life Plan*

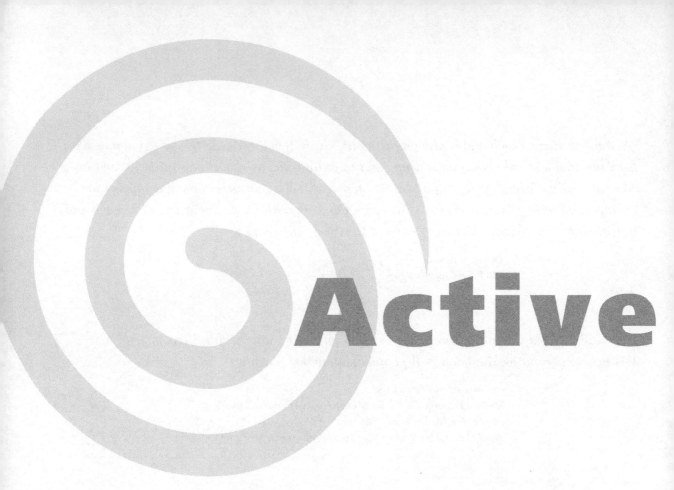

Active

NEWLY UPDATED *

Wellness™

Feel Good for Life

Gayle Reichler, M.S., R.D., CDN

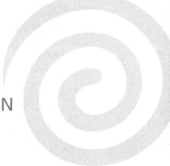

AVERY • A MEMBER OF PENGUIN GROUP (USA) INC.

To Doug for his love, support, and belief in my mission.

**To my clients, whose efforts to strive
for optimum health, increased self-awareness,
and growth in their lives are a continual inspiration.**

a member of
Penguin Group (USA) Inc.
375 Hudson Street
New York, NY 10014
www.penguin.com

Copyright © 1998, 2003 by Gayle Reichler
Published in hard cover by Time-Life Custom Publishing
Line art by Alfred Giuliani

Library of Congress Cataloging-in-Publication Data
Reichler, Gayle.
    Active wellness : feel good for life / Gayle Reichler.
      p.   cm.
    "Newly updated."
    Previous ed. was published with subtitle: A personalized 10 step program for healthy body, mind & spirit.
    Includes bibliographical references and index.
    ISBN 1-58333-169-7
    1. Health.   2. Nutrition.   3. Exercise.   4. Stress management.   I. Title.
RA776.9.R435   2003   2003056250
613—dc21

Printed in the United States of America
10 9 8 7 6 5 4 3 2 1

BOOK DESIGN BY TANYA MAIBORODA

Acknowledgments

THE REALIZATION OF a vision requires love, respect, attention, and time. Translating Active Wellness, the program, into *Active Wellness,* a healthy and vital book, required all this and more. Each person involved in Active Wellness has made an important contribution to the book you hold in your hands. Although this list will seem comprehensive, I will not be able to mention everyone. Therefore, I would first like to thank all those who have been a part of Active Wellness and who have contributed to its development.

Active Wellness, the book, evolved from my meeting Paula Glaser, whose belief and enthusiasm became the catalyst that helped launch this project. Our fortuitous meeting led me to Dorie Simmonds, my literary agent. Dorie's tremendous expertise made it possible for the paperback book to become a reality by finding it a home at Penguin Group.

I applaud the dynamic team at Avery, Penguin Group. Every step toward producing the final version of this book has been done with professionalism, creativity, and wisdom. A writer couldn't ask for more. I am looking forward to publishing the next book, a cookbook to follow *Active Wellness*. I feel very fortunate to be working with everyone at Penguin: John Duff, publisher, for his vision, foresight, expertise, and leadership; Eileen Bertelli, executive editor and director of sales, for her talent in coordinating her two specialties together so very well. Eileen's spirit and hard work were powerful driving forces that helped me to strive to excel at all the tasks at hand in revising *Active Wellness* for its paperback debut. Thank you also to those behind the scenes—the copy editors, line editors, proofreaders, designers, marketers, and publicist Eric Levine, for being ready for the media and taking initiative. For my picture, a big thank-you to friend and photographer John Stuart, who always makes me feel confident, because he strives for the perfect shot every time.

To everyone who took the time to provide a quote or picture for the book, I thank you. The book would not have been the same without your contributions: Ann, Jennifer, Sallyann, Ed, Larry, Fran, Susan, Elaine, Laurie, and Lisa. And to those I work with closely through my counseling and group Active Wellness Program and at Avon Salon and Spa and Avon Wellness, thank you for your continued support and promotion of the program.

To those who have inspired me and served as my teachers and supporters: Sharron Dalton, R.D., Ph.D.; Carol Guber; Dr. James Kennedy; Marion Nestle, Ph.D., M.P.H.; Dr. Dean Ornish; Marilyn Majchrzak, R.D.; Lisa Powell, R.D.; and Susan Bishop and Alice Austin at the American Heart Association, New York City.

A thank-you to all the others who have contributed to *Active Wellness* through their effort and support of the program and the book, including Amy Beim; Amie Hoffman, R.D.; Wendi Daniels; and Kathleen Flaherty. A special thank-you to Dr. James Kennedy, who found my cancer, and who continues to provide quality care for both my family and me. And to those who are invaluable for their ongoing love and support of all that I do, my family and friends.

Contents

Author's Note

THE ACTIVE WELLNESS PROGRAM is an adjunct to, not a substitute for, conventional medical therapy. It can be considered part of your preventive medical program. The nutrition, fitness, and stress-management plans discussed in this book are recommendations by a Registered Dietitian. Before you start your program, it is important that you consult with your physician and other health-care providers.

I also recommend that you maintain routine medical care and monitor your condition as you proceed in the Active Wellness Program. It is also important that you do not stop taking or make changes in any of your medications without first consulting with your prescribing physician.

One goal of this book is to make you aware of the impact of healthy lifestyle options on your overall well-being. More specifically, I want to help you learn how to reach your personal health goals through satisfying behavioral changes. To that end, this book will introduce you to the strengths of the allied health fields of nutrition, exercise physiology, psychology, and alternative health practices such as yoga. Since many of you will be trying these health practices for the first time, please feel free to contact Active Wellness with any questions you may have. If you are unsure about whether the recommendations in this book are right for you, please contact your health-care provider. You can contact Active Wellness directly online at www.activewellness.com.

Introduction and My Story

CONGRATULATIONS! You've just discovered Active Wellness, a flexible, easy-to-follow program that will provide you with the keys to achieve your weight and health goals. As you gear up to begin, the first step is to believe that you will succeed—and that you will look and feel better and younger than you have in years! If you've tried other weight-loss programs that haven't worked, don't despair. You *will* succeed with Active Wellness!

The Active Wellness Program works because it's not a diet—it's an energizing, satisfying, healthy way of living that you create to fit your lifestyle. If you are a mother at home, your Active Wellness Program will work with your schedule, just as it will work for someone who is in their thirties and working long hours or someone in their sixties facing retirement. With Active Wellness, you have a blueprint from which you create a personalized program to meet your goals. By taking the whole being into account—mind, body, and spirit—Active Wellness gives you a total approach to health that works for life.

On your journey to good health, you'll have my support as your wellness coach every step of the way. I will give you the tools you need to conquer old habits and the strategies to create the new healthy behaviors you desire. You will get sensible, realistic recommendations that are easy to integrate into your daily routine. Each day, you will nurture yourself with appetizing menus, a flexible exercise routine, and simple stress-reduction techniques—an entire program based on your preferences. You will never feel exhausted or deprived!

You don't have to pay expensive spa prices or hire a personal trainer. Active Wellness will provide you with everything you need to become your own best wellness coach. Plus, you will have the support of www.activewellness.com for any questions you have during your program.

The confusion you may have about what exactly is a healthy diet will be resolved, because you will learn what is right for you with a program that is based on medical research. You can overcome obstacles that have frustrated you for years, such as craving junk food, struggling with stress overload, or never finding time in your hectic schedule to exercise. Within just a few weeks you'll see results, whether it's a five-pound weight loss, newfound energy, or a sense of control over your schedule. If improved health is your primary concern, you may find that you can reduce your blood-pressure medication, control your cholesterol, improve your osteoporosis, or manage your diabetes more easily.

The Active Wellness Program doesn't end when you lose that extra twenty pounds or complete your first 10K walk. Instead, it encourages you to continually reevaluate yourself in order to make your new healthy behaviors last a lifetime.

The seven steps of Active Wellness set you up with the strategies you need to feel good for life, so you can attain your ideal weight, increase your energy, and reduce your stress. The seven steps include:

Step 1: Mentally Preparing Yourself for the Wellness Journey
Step 2: Forming New Healthy Habits and Conquering Triggers That Sabotage Your Success
Step 3: Getting Started with Your Personal Eating Plan
Step 4: Putting Your Eating Plan into Practice Anywhere
Step 5: Your Personal Physical Fitness Plan

Step 6: Ways to Manage Stress
Step 7: Maintaining Active Wellness for a Lifetime

You won't fail with Active Wellness, because the program allows you to achieve your goals at your own pace. Regardless of your lifestyle obstacles—whether you travel a lot for business or are always busy with your children—you will learn how to set goals that help you make time for yourself and your healthy-lifestyle program. In return, you'll have the energy you need to live life at your absolute best. I've done it, and I've helped thousands of others reach their goals. Now it's *your* turn!

But before we start the program, I'd like to share my personal story about how I came to create Active Wellness.

My Story

From an early age, I struggled with my weight. At one point, I gained twenty-five pounds in a year. I'll never forget how big I felt—and how unhealthy. All I wanted was to fit into my clothes and feel attractive again. I tried many diets, including the Scarsdale Diet and Weight Watchers, yet I always regained the weight I'd lost. I knew there had to be a better way. In search of a plan that would enable me to maintain a healthy weight without giving up my favorite foods, I began to study nutrition. My newfound knowledge helped me lose weight, and now I would be able to help people learn the truth about how to achieve their ideal weight *and* eat well!

Everything seemed to be going my way. It was late fall of 1991, and I was winding down my graduate studies at New York University and looking forward to my new career as a nutritionist, chef, and health-care counselor. As the last golden days of autumn appeared in New York, I was filled with excitement and optimism about the future. Little did I know that my life was about to change in ways I never could have imagined.

After pulling my back playing tennis, I went to my doctor for a checkup. He was always very thorough and sent me to have some tests on my thyroid, which seemed enlarged. One test led to another, and before I knew it I was back in the doctor's office to hear my diagnosis: I had thyroid cancer. I was shocked!

Me? Cancer? A young, healthy, active woman? How could this be? My doctor informed me that my thyroid would have to be removed, along with any other cancerous tissue in my neck. I left my doctor's office that morning feeling overwhelmed. I realized how much I valued each day. I not only wanted to live, *I wanted to live more healthfully*. I didn't know why I had gotten cancer, but I was sure as heck determined to do what I could so that it never came back in any other form.

I'm convinced that almost any problem can be managed with the right attitude, the right tools, and a lot of determination. I saw my cancer as a physical challenge and an emotional wake-up call. It was on the eve of my surgery, in the quiet of my hospital room, that I had the first of many epiphanies about what I needed to do. I had to make every day count toward my new goal of optimal health for me and ultimately for those I hoped to teach. I named this new mission "Active Wellness."

By the time I left the hospital, I was physically sick and emotionally drained. The radiation treatment left my body feeling assaulted and polluted. I was also beginning to experience other side effects. Since the thyroid regulates metabolism, and I no longer had one, I couldn't produce the hormone that regulates weight. As a result, extra pounds started to appear. Both my memory and my thinking became sluggish. I was twenty-eight, but I felt more than twice my age. My doctor put me on thyroid medication, but I needed something more. Determined to feel healthy again, I resumed a simple healthy eating and exercise program. Then I set out to learn all there was to know about achieving optimal health.

It was the early nineties, when the word *wellness* was not commonly used in our vocabulary, and the study of complementary medicine did not exist as a recognized field. Yet there were several businesses on the cutting edge of knowledge in health and healing, so I went to work for them. I was a nutritionist at the Canyon Ranch Spa, which offers numerous services, including behavioral therapy, alternative medicine, and cutting-edge medical testing, and I worked alongside Dean Ornish, M.D., the author of the best-selling book *Reversing Heart Disease,* which explains how lifestyle change can heal an unhealthy heart and unclog your arteries. In my quest to learn what works, I tried as many practices as I could, including acupuncture, biofeedback, yoga, meditation, and classes in Chinese and Aruvyedic medicine, both practices based on balancing the energy fields in your body, one Asian and one Indian in orientation.

At that point, I realized I had missed a *huge* piece of the wellness equation. While eating well and maintaining a regular exercise schedule are important, something more is required. In order to gain control of your weight and health, you need to address *all* aspects of your well-being: mind, body, and spirit. My goal became clear—to create a program that provides the tools and structure you need to reach your optimal level of wellness.

Through research, practice, and some great fun, the Active Wellness Program began. I am happy to say that thirteen years after my initial diagnosis of cancer, I have reached my ultimate goal: Because of the Active Wellness Program I am happy, healthy, and strong. Practicing each part of my program every day allows me to live at my peak level of wellness.

As your "wellness coach," my job is to help you take charge of your health by providing options on which to base your new lifestyle. You then create a nutritious eating program based on foods you enjoy, an exercise program that matches your fitness level, and a plan to reduce stress. With Active Wellness, you'll learn how easy it can be to take care of yourself once you know what your body needs.

Active Wellness will guide you as you create an effective plan designed to deliver results. The program recognizes your individual health goals and celebrates the fact that the path traveled to ideal weight and optimal health is as unique as the travelers themselves.

If you follow my lead and practice each part of the Active Wellness Program, you'll reach your goal, whether it's weight loss, lower cholesterol or blood pressure, or better control of diabetes. The first step is to believe that you will succeed. With your new Active Wellness blueprint in hand, results can be yours in just a few weeks. Before you know it, you will be on your way to reaching your goals and living at your personal best.

During times of challenge and when you have questions, you can seek support and advice online via my web site, www.activewellness.com.

May the journey be as richly rewarding and exhilarating for you as it has been for me.

—GAYLE REICHLER, M.S., R.D., CDN
Wellness Coach

1

Mentally Preparing Yourself for the Wellness Journey

THE FIRST STEP in your Active Wellness journey is to believe you will succeed in achieving your health and weight goals and that you will feel better than you have felt in *years*. Active Wellness is not just another "diet"; it is a sound program, based on scientific and medical research on eating, exercise, and stress management. Founded on the principle that living a healthy lifestyle needs to be satisfying, Active Wellness's goal is to provide you with the tools you need to create a healthy lifestyle you will enjoy. Now, instead of just wishing for good health and ideal weight, you have Active Wellness to progress you to your goals.

Getting started requires the critical first step of taking time to mentally prepare yourself for your Active Wellness journey. Every successful endeavor first begins in the mind as an idea, a thought, a dream, a conviction. As any great athlete, entrepreneur, or performer will tell you, "You can't do it if your head's not in it." You also can't do it if you don't know where you're going, or why, or how you're going to get there. Many well-intentioned people have set out to make great changes or accomplish a singular task, only to give up in the early stages because their goals and methods were unfocused, unrealistic, or simply impossible. Pursuing wellness is no different than pursuing any goal—except that it may be the most important goal you ever pursue.

As you begin your Active Wellness journey, you need to be crystal clear about what you want to achieve for yourself and how you're going to get it. This chapter is about helping you find that mental clarity and mapping out a strategy for success.

Your strategy will be based on the small Active Wellness steps you will be taking each day that, when accumulated, will lead you easily and successfully to your ultimate goals. The participants who achieve the best results in the Active Wellness Program are those who set some time aside on a consistent basis to practice their program.

Whether reading this book, restocking your pantry with healthy foods, creating a meal plan, walking a mile, doing a stretching routine, lifting weights, or exploring stress-reduction techniques, you will want to carve out twenty to thirty minutes a day for your Active Wellness. The sooner you devote the time, the sooner you will see results; and the sooner you see results, the more encouraged you will be to stick with your program. As your wellness coach, I will provide you with new information in each chapter that will help you change unhealthy behaviors into healthy lifetime habits. Once you are ready to devote attention to your health and well-being, the next step is to determine how you want to look and feel when you achieve your ultimate goal.

Envisioning a New You

Take a moment, close your eyes, and conjure up a magnificent vision of yourself. This vision is not only everything you have always *wanted* to be, but everything you were always meant to be, radiant with health, energy, and confidence on your own unique terms. Guard this vision and hold it close to your heart. It is the reason you picked up this book and have started the Active Wellness journey. It is your motivation for the effort required to change. It is your impetus for starting down the wellness path as well as your reward for successfully completing the journey. Who will that new you be?

A strong mental image of how you want to look and feel at the end of the Active Wellness journey can be a great motivating tool as you progress through each step of your training program. Asking yourself some pointed questions will help you clarify the vision of yourself that you want to see. Often, the answers reflect what you'd like to change about your current health, appearance, and lifestyle. Active Wellness participants in my classes have asked themselves the following questions:

Will I be thinner?
Will I feel more confident?
Will I lower my cholesterol?
Will I have my blood sugar under control?
Will I feel less stressed?
Will I be happier?
Will I have more energy?
Will I walk up a flight of stairs without feeling winded?
Will I wear that suit I bought last year that I can't fit into now?

Ask yourself these questions or come up with new ones that are relevant for you. Then turn these questions into answers, into strong, active, and confident statements of belief. These answers, and beliefs, form your Active Wellness vision. The more vivid and clear your images, the more successful you will be in achieving them. Below are some sample Active Wellness images from individuals who have used the program.

I have more energy.
I am stronger.
I am leaner.
I am medication free.
I am easily jogging three miles.
I am radiating joy and good health.

Now create some Active Wellness images that are uniquely yours. What do you want to achieve from the Active Wellness Program? Think of the above questions that you asked yourself, and turn some of those questions into vivid and positive answers. It can be helpful to write out your vision, because we tend to go toward a path that is visible and clearly defined. You can record your vision in the space below or on a note card.

Your Vision

_____

_____

_____

_____

_____

These are the images to carry in your mind's eye throughout the Active Wellness Program. They are your visual goals. To help you stay focused on your vision, carry your list of images in your pocket or post them on your refrigerator door or in your calendar at your office. Share them with friends and family and ask them for support.

Planning Your Goals

Now that you have a clear mental and written vision of the person you want to be at the end of your Active Wellness journey, you probably also have an idea of what you need to do to attain your vision. Now is the time to reframe that idea into clear and realistic long- and short-term goals that will help you define your focus of the Active Wellness Program. Your goals will put your ideal vision into a plan and will provide targets for you to work toward.

First, establish a primary, or long-term, health goal that encompasses the vision you are trying to achieve. This also becomes your main health objective. Similar to your vision of a new you, your long-term health goal drives your entire Active Wellness Program and urges you toward success. Your long-term goal is the ultimate achievement you are committed to realizing as a result of your efforts.

Examples of common and realistic long-term goals are:

* Losing ten pounds
* Lowering cholesterol in eight weeks
* Establishing a routine fitness program three days a week

* Normalizing blood sugars
* Managing stress

You may choose to make your long-term goal more detailed and individual, such as wanting to fit into a smaller size pair of pants or being able to stop taking blood-pressure medication. If weight loss is what you desire, make sure your goal is motivating enough for you. Many times losing weight for the sake of being thinner isn't enough to motivate us to take action. Often what motivates us is something more personal, such as being able to walk up the stairs without getting out of breath or wanting to feel more in control of our actions.

Do remember to tackle only one long-term goal at a time. You don't want to become overwhelmed by taking on too much or defeat your good intentions before you even have a chance to start your wellness journey. Trust your instincts about how far you need to go to realize the vision of a new you. Most people have an innate sense about what they can achieve for themselves in terms of their health.

Next are your short-term goals that help you progress during your program. Your short-term goal can be thought of as something good you do for

FOR WRITING EFFECTIVE GOALS

- *State your goal in the positive*—it will turn your attention to the future.
- *The goal needs to be realistic and within your power to achieve*—always remember to set yourself up for success. When you achieve your initial goal, you can always make a new goal.
- *Make it visible and measurable*—so you know when you achieve it.

yourself every day and every week that makes your life easier and more consistent with your goals. It is not something you feel you "should" be doing, but something you want to do to further your goal. Think of short-term goals as the "the baby steps," or small victories that lead you to your ultimate goal and vision. One of the best ways to move forward is to conquer one short-term goal at a time. When your short-term goals become automatic, it is easier to manage your health and your weight. You can choose to write down daily goals or weekly goals. For example, if your long-term goal is weight loss, your short-term goals for the week might be to walk thirty minutes every evening, or eat two fruits a day instead of desserts, or have one sweet instead of two each day. In this scenario, you are not only losing weight, you are becoming physically fit, lowering your fat intake, and probably your cholesterol at the same time, and taking preventive measures against heart disease and cancer. You are well on your way to achieving your long-term goal of weight loss along with optimum wellness.

It is important to set realistic short-term goals so you can succeed with one and move on to the next. Therefore, you can choose to have only one goal of the week instead of two or three. Many of my clients find that if their schedule is hectic, they can only devote energy to one short-term goal a week, because it would be overwhelming to do more. I want you to succeed at your goals each week; therefore, be sure to make them achievable. If a goal is too lofty, it can set you up for defeat, inhibiting your success with the program.

Below are some examples of effective—and ineffective—words and phrases for framing your short-term goals.

Effectively Phrased Goals

* I will increase (the number of vegetables I eat).
* I will reduce (my fat intake/my alcohol intake).
* I will eliminate (junk food).
* I will limit (my sweets/my caffeine intake).
* I will add (more fruits to my diet).

Ineffectively Phrased Goals

* I want to be thin.
* I have to control my cholesterol and blood pressure.
* I must de-stress.

Writing your goals is an important step in acknowledging them more concretely. It underscores your desire to achieve them. The more your goals match your actions, the better you will feel about the program and, more important, about yourself. When creating your short-term goals, keep your weekly schedule in mind and decide on a goal that makes sense in your life that week. Use your calendar to write in a time when you plan to work on your weekly goal. Think of the time you set aside for your Active Wellness Program as an appointment you can't break. It is important to make yourself and your program a number-one priority so you can achieve your goals.

There are long- and short-term goal charts on page 9. Take a moment now to fill them in with your initial long- and short-term goals. Additional Goal Charts can be found in the appendix.

Testimonial

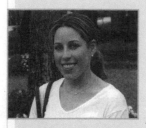

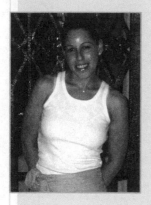

I started the Active Wellness Program because I was eager to lose weight and get in better shape for my wedding. Plus, I was tired of not having energy and feeling stuck in unhealthy eating routines that were not helping me reach my goal. My fiancé and I were constantly grabbing meals on the go and having late dinners, trying to juggle work and planning our wedding. I was skeptical that Active Wellness was going to help me, because I am such a picky eater I can count the types of food I like to eat on two hands. I had seen too many brides diet incorrectly and look sickly on their wedding day, and I didn't want to have to resort to an unhealthy program. I came to know Active Wellness through friends who had a healthy-lifestyle approach. I looked to Active Wellness to help me feel my best for my big day.

My goal was to lose ten pounds and trim down at least one dress size. The first step was to understand the approach and look at what and how I was eating. Using the Active Wellness Program, I began tracking the foods I was eating. I quickly realized that I was consuming a lot of protein and sugar and not too much else. With the guidance of the Active Wellness Program, I created a balanced eating routine of foods I enjoyed and foods I could easily find while on the go working and planning my wedding. I couldn't believe that, even with the limited selection of foods I liked, I could create a satisfying eating plan filled with nutrients and lean calories. Soon after I changed my eating, my energy started to pick up. Active Wellness also directed me toward an exercise routine for my body type and activity level. The weight came off slowly, but before I knew it I had dropped two sizes and created a plan that I could use even after the wedding was over. I was thrilled. I looked exactly the way I wanted walking down the aisle!

© *Jennifer, age twenty-eight, lost 12 pounds and 2 dress sizes*

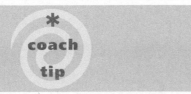

Do your goals coincide with a personal value? The more a goal honors a value, or what you hold to be important, the more motivated you will be to achieve your goal and the less you will have to come up against your list of "shoulds." Think about how it might feel to follow a goal you didn't hold to be important—most likely you wouldn't find the energy to devote effort to achieving it. Examples of some values are: health, accomplishment, commitment, humor, joy, trust, learning, accuracy, spirituality, integrity. What do you value, and how does this help you achieve your Active Wellness goal?

Goal Chart

Long-Term Goals

_____

_____

_____

_____

_____

Short-Term Goals

_____

_____

_____

_____

_____

Assessing Your Personal Health History and Lifestyle

Both the Personal Health History and the Lifestyle Assessment include medical and nutrition assessments that significantly affect your personalized well-

A Note on Cholesterol and Triglycerides

If you haven't had your cholesterol and triglycerides checked in over a year, or if you don't know the types of cholesterol, I recommend that you contact your doctor. Compare the numbers with the acceptable ranges listed in the chart below. Please note whether your numbers are high, low, or normal. Then fill in your results in questions 2 and 3 in Personal Health History.

Recommended Cholesterol and Triglyceride Levels

Cholesterol	In mg/dl	Risk Level
Total Cholesterol:	≤200	Desirable
	200–220	Borderline High
	>220	High
Low-**D**ensity Lipoprotein (**Least D**esirable)		
(LDL Cholesterol):	<100	Desirable
	<130	Near Desirable
	130–159	Borderline High
	≥160	High
High-**D**ensity Lipoprotein (**Highly D**esirable)		
(HDL Cholesterol):	<40	Low
	36–59	Near Desirable
	≥60	Desirable
Total Cholesterol/HDL Ratio:	<3	Desirable
	3–4	Borderline High
	>4	High
Triglycerides:	<150	Desirable
	150–199	Borderline High
	200–499	High
	>500	Very High

Note: These numbers are based on fasting triglycerides.

ness plan and therefore your long- and short-term goals. You may want to modify your short-term health goals after assessing your personal health and lifestyle.

Answer the questions on pages 11 to 14. Write your answers in the spaces provided, so you will have a record of your health history and lifestyle at the beginning of your Active Wellness Program. As you answer each question, record the points that correspond to your answers on a separate piece of paper. At the end of the Personal Health History and the Lifestyle Assessment, tally your points. This information will determine your needs for the Active Wellness Program.

Personal Health History

1 Do you have any of the following?

a. Elevated blood pressure: ____Yes (0 points) ____No (5 points)

b. Uncontrolled blood sugar: ____Yes (0 points) ____No (5 points)

c. Osteopenia or osteoporosis: _____Yes (0 points) _____No (5 points)

d. Cancer of any type: _____Yes (0 points) _____No (5 points)

Cancer in remission: _____Yes (2 points)

e. Between 5 and 30 lbs of weight to lose: _____ (2 points)

<5 lbs of weight to lose: ___ (5 points)

>30 lbs of weight to lose: ____ (0 points)

2 Does your family (your biological parents and siblings) health history include any of the following health issues?

a. High cholesterol: Yes ___ (0 points) No ____ (3 points)

b. High blood pressure: Yes ___ (0 points) No ____ (3 points)

c. Diabetes or hypoglycemia: Yes ___ (0 points) No ____ (3 points)

d. Cancer: Yes ___ (0 points) No ____ (3 points)

e. Osteoporosis: Yes ___ (0 points) No ____ (3 points)

3 What are your current cholesterol and triglyceride levels?

a. Total cholesterol: ____ (If >200 mg/dl, give yourself 0 points; if your levels are <200, give yourself 5 points.)

b. Your HDL (highly desirable) cholesterol: ____ (If <40 mg/dl, give yourself 0 points; if your levels are >40, give yourself 5 points.)

c. Your LDL (least desirable) cholesterol: _____ (If >130 mg/dl, give yourself 0 points; if your levels are <130, give yourself 5 points.)

d. Your triglycerides: _____ (If >200 mg/dl, give yourself 0 points; if your levels are >150, give yourself 5 points.)

4 Do you take a multivitamin every day?

___ No (0 points) ____Sometimes (3 points) ___ Yes (5 points)

5 Do you take a supplement containing omega-3 fats daily or eat fish three or more times a week?

___ No (0 points) ____Sometimes (3 points) ___ Yes (5 points)

6 Alcohol intake:_____ drinks per day

(Use the following point scale for alcohol: 0 to 1 drink/day = 5 points; 2 to 3 drinks/day = 2 points; 3 to 5 drinks/day = 0 points.)

7 Tobacco intake: _____ nonsmoker (5 points)

_____ quit smoking (3 points)

_____ smoker (0 points)

_____ chewing tobacco (0 points)

8 Exercise:

If your exercise routine includes:

a. _____ Aerobic exercise

0 times/week	(0 points)
1 to 2 times/week	(3 points)
3 to 4 times/week	(5 points)

b. _____ Strength training

0 times/week	(0 points)
1 time/week	(2 points)
2 times/week	(4 points)
3 or more times/week	(5 points)

c. _____ Stretching exercise

        0 times/week   (0 points)

        1 to 2 times/week   (2 points)

        3 to 4 times/week   (4 points)

        Every day   (5 points)

PERSONAL HEALTH HISTORY SUBTOTAL: _____

Lifestyle Assessment

1 Over the course of a week, how would you describe your overall energy level? Rate your energy level based on the scale listed below. At one end of the spectrum is "Full of Pep" (5 points), and at the other is "Exhausted" (1 point). Circle the number on the continuum that indicates how you feel most of the time:

Full of Pep   5 4 3 2 1   Exhausted

2 Over the course of a week, how would you describe your overall stress level? Rate your stress level based on the scale listed below. At one end of the spectrum you are "Stress Free," as if you were relaxing on a vacation with no worries. At the other extreme is "Highly Stressed"—you are at the end of your rope and about to blow a fuse. Three is neutral. Pick the place on the continuum that describes how you most often feel during the course of a week:

Stress Free   5 4 3 2 1   Highly Stressed

3 How well do you sleep?

_____ I almost always get the amount of sleep I need; I rarely feel tired. (5 points)

_____ I feel tired because I usually fall short of enough sleep by a few hours a night. (2 points)

_____ I never get the amount of sleep I need, and I am always tired. (0 points)

4 When you eat, are you:

    a. Eating on the run?

        ____ Yes (0 points)

        ____ No (5 points)

        ____ Sometimes (2 points)

    b. Eating when you're not hungry?

        ____ Yes (0 points)

        ____ No (5 points)

        ____ Sometimes (2 points)

5 When you eat, do you:

    a. Eat quickly (finish your meal within 10 to 15 minutes)?

        ____ Yes (0 points)

        ____ No (5 points)

        ____ Sometimes (2 points)

    b. Skip meals?

        ____ Yes (0 points)

        ____ No (5 points)

        ____ Sometimes (2 points)

    c. Eat late (after 9:00 P.M.)?

        ____ Yes (0 points)

        ____ No (5 points)

        ____ Sometimes (2 points)

_____ LIFESTYLE ASSESSMENT SUBTOTAL

_____ PERSONAL HEALTH HISTORY AND LIFESTYLE ASSESSMENT TOTAL

When you tally the total points in your Personal Health History and Lifestyle Assessment, you get a good picture of how well you are living an Active Wellness lifestyle:

If your score is 135, you are doing an excellent job at maintaining Active Wellness and can use the program to achieve an even better level of optimal mind/body/spirit health.

If your score is 114 to 134, you have some room for improvement. Use the Active Wellness Program as your guide to incorporate the changes you need in order to achieve your optimal level of health and well-being.

If your score is 76 to 114, you are not doing very well at living an Active Wellness lifestyle, and you are putting yourself at risk for further health complications. By following the Active Wellness Program you can greatly improve your health status and quality of life.

If your score is 2 to 75, you are leading a lifestyle of high risk. You will feel healthier as you progress in your Active Wellness Program. By following the program you can improve your chances of reducing disease risks. The lower the numbers in the categories above, the greater your health risks.

Genetic Influences

The personal assessment you've just completed gives you a clear indication of where you are vulnerable or at high risk because of your current medical conditions and lifestyle choices. By looking at your family health history, you will be able to draw some general conclusions about what types of diseases can be inherited from your family gene pool. Diseases that appear in our adult years can occur when genes we inherited from our family members are triggered by a variety of environmental factors—some within our control, such as diet, stress, and unhealthy behaviors, and some beyond our control, such as environmental factors. With Active Wellness you can enhance your quality of life by creating a healthy lifestyle program that will help keep your body young, fit, and healthy, giving you the best chance of feeling your best for life.

Staying on Track During Each Step of the Program

As your coach, I will encourage you and provide you with useful information in each new step. I will teach you new and innovative ways to eat healthfully. I will show you how to balance your meals for optimum nutrition and energy, how to incorporate a variety of physical-fitness routines into your life, how to practice stress-reduction techniques, and how to change unhealthy behaviors into healthy lifetime habits.

But only you can bring the critically important ingredients of motivation and commitment. One of the ways you can keep up your level of commitment and motivation is to be mindful of the "three Ps"—Practice, Pacing, and Patience—throughout your program.

Practice: By practicing new Active Wellness skills every day, they eventually become second nature to you and empower you to master more new steps, routines, and behaviors.

Pacing: Every moment toward a healthy change or healthy habit is progress. But some changes come slowly, with more difficulty. Expect that some changes will take you time. The steps are meant to be incremental and cumulative. Your focus is on making small changes and short-term, attainable goals. As you progress through the program, the small changes accumulate and lead you to large changes and more complex goals. Eventually, you reach the point where Active Wellness has affected not only your health and weight but also your self-esteem, courage, and confidence.

Patience: Above all, be patient with yourself. However slowly and steadily you are moving, remember that you are probably confronting a lifetime of unhealthy behaviors. Don't despair. Forgive yourself and just move on. Sooner than you think, you can be enjoying one success after another. Just remember—always stick with it. If you take your time, you will succeed with your goals.

If you remain focused on reaching your goals, you will get there. During your Active Wellness journey, you will be introduced to new foods, new behaviors, and new lifestyles. You will begin to view your life with an Active Wellness perspective, and you will feel better and happier in mind, body, and spirit. I guarantee it. Congratulations! You have now completed Step 1, and you are on your way to achieving Active Wellness. Now, it's time to move on to Step 2—learning how to change unwanted habits!

Main Points to Mentally Preparing Yourself for the Wellness Journey

✔ Believe you will succeed in achieving your weight and health goals.

✔ Determine how you want to look and feel when you reach your ultimate wellness goals.

✔ List your ultimate goal and the small steps (short-term goals) you know will help you get there.

✔ Check in with yourself and make sure you have realistic expectations.

✔ Take the Active Wellness Personal Health History and Lifestyle Assessment to assess your current state of well-being.

✔ Use the three Ps—Practice, Pacing, and Patience—to help you stay on track during each step of your program.

✔ If you have questions, email Active Wellness at www.activewellness.com.

Forming New Healthy Habits and Conquering Triggers That Sabotage Your Success

OFTEN IN LIFE we find that our goals, dreams, and opportunities are sabotaged, not by outside forces but by ourselves. We may start each day with the best of intentions only to be sidetracked by old, unhealthy habits that get in the way of our success. You might have a particularly hard week at work, have plans for a big family event, or be faced with a series of stressful situations.

Even seemingly innocuous behaviors can become obstacles to our success—always having coffee with breakfast or a sugary treat in the late afternoon, never sitting down to savor a meal, or constantly working until there is no time left for exercise in your day. Whatever it is, you may unexpectedly hit the proverbial brick wall along your path to good health, suddenly reverting back to old habits that, while comfortable, do not serve your goals.

Long-established habitual routines may seem like natural patterns in your life, but are they helping you or hurting you? If some of your habitual behaviors are preventing you from living a healthy life or enjoying a healthy self-image, they are definitely hurting you. Now is the time to develop strategies for changing old behaviors into new healthy habits. This chapter will teach you how to do that, beginning with a look at how habits are formed, followed by a discussion of the tools you can use to change them.

The Habit Chain—How It's Formed and How It Can Be Broken

By taking this step at the beginning of your Active Wellness Program, you will be equipped with the knowledge you need to prevent your old habits from

SUCCESSFUL INGREDIENTS FOR CHANGE

Creating new healthy habits can be one of the most effective ways you can improve your health. One small change repeated consistently often leads to big results.

The ingredients needed to make successful change include:

1. Developing an awareness of the behavior you want to change.
2. Knowledge of the tools you can use to make healthy changes.
3. The motivation and determination to choose an Active Wellness coaching tool to help you make the change, and the fortitude to do your best to be consistent in maintaining your new healthier behavior until it becomes a habit.
4. An understanding that ingrained behaviors that get in the way of your new healthy lifestyle take time to change. It is important to give yourself a chance and not be too hard on yourself. Trust that you are doing the best you can. It takes time for our brain to remember and record a new action into a habit. The new behavior will take hold eventually. So be patient with yourself and don't give up.

interfering with your goals. The tools in this step will teach you how to take emotional control of personal situations instead of allowing them to control you. Like a painter who has a palette of colors to choose from, you will have a selection of tools and responses to use for various situations. You will see how empowering it can be to choose actions that are consistent with your goals, avoiding the obstacles that typically can get in the way. Before you know it, your short-term goals will be easy successes and you will be well on your way to achieving your ultimate goals for weight and wellness!

Habits are acquired behavior patterns that are regularly repeated over time until they become nearly involuntary or unconscious actions in our everyday lives. A habit is the end result of a chain of events.

The sidebar illustrates the habit chain. The first link is a triggering event or circumstance that acts like an ignition and starts the chain reaction. Once a triggering event occurs, we react and respond in the form of thoughts, followed by feelings. As a result of our thoughts and feelings, we take action. The more often we use a particular action to cope with our thoughts and feelings, the more likely it is to develop into a habit.

Many habits are good and constructive for our health—exercising regularly, taking vitamins, and brushing one's teeth are just a few examples. Unfortunately, many other habits are bad for our health. Often, these are habits that we develop as coping mechanisms for negative or uncomfortable feelings and events. These coping habits too often work against our goals for good health, including smoking when we are stressed, drinking too much when we are wired up, or overeating when we are depressed. When you understand each link in the habit chain, you can learn how to interrupt the chain of events and end unhealthy habits.

Event

The triggering event that starts the chain reaction that leads to a particular habit may be significant or insignificant. It can be a serious emotional trigger, such as an argument with a loved one, or a banal event, such as walking past a bakery. Like a catalyst in a chemical reaction, a triggering event is a stimulus that ignites a change in our behavior. On page 22 there is a list of common triggers that many Active Wellness participants have identified as obstacles on their own wellness journeys. See if any of these ring true for you.

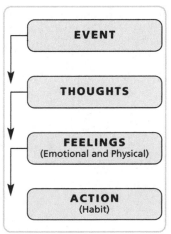

Thoughts

Once a trigger or circumstance occurs that ignites our thoughts, we begin a conversation with ourselves that stress experts and psychologists call "self-talk."

For example, reading this book may be triggering self-talk in your head. Perhaps you are thinking, "I don't believe this program will work for me. It may work for other people, but not for me." This is a typical kind of negative self-talk, and it almost always leads to defeat when you are trying to change specific behaviors and habits. The talk is not even rooted in fact but is merely an assumption, probably based on past "failures" that came about because of the negative self-talk. The truth is, you don't know what works for you unless you give it a try. And any attempt to change, no matter how small, is never a failure, but always a positive step forward. A more empowering type of self-talk when facing the challenge of changing unhealthy habits is, "This just might work for me. I can certainly give it my best effort."

SELF-TALK

The easiest place to break a link in the habit chain is with your thoughts. When you change your thought, a cascade of changes will follow down your habit chain, ultimately helping you change your old habit. Changing your self-talk can help you take more positive action, because new thoughts generate new feelings, which in turn can translate into different, healthier responses.

You are in control of the self-talk you choose to listen to and choose to believe. As you learn to change your self-talk, you'll need to acknowledge the original negative thought and change it to a positive thought. "Listen" for your self-talk; we talk to ourselves hundreds of times a day, but do we recognize the self-talk that leads to undesired actions or bad habits? What kinds of things do you say to yourself? Are they invariably negative or positive? What emotional feelings and physical sensations accompany those thoughts?

Words that can help you identify negative self-talk include *can't, won't, shouldn't, never,* and *not.* Positive, proactive, and transformational words include *can, will, want, should, always,* and *I am.* Using Tom's story, below, as an example, you can see how Tom changed his thoughts and feelings to transform an old habit into a new healthy one.

Tom's Story: An Active Wellness client who was trying to lose weight, Tom frequently put in extra hours at the office. When this happened, his thoughts were, "I hate that I have to work late. They are not paying me enough for all the hours I put in." The event—having to work late—triggered negative thoughts. Those thoughts, in turn, triggered negative emotional and physical feelings. The negative feelings then led Tom to engage in a self-destructive habit.

In this case, Tom's thoughts caused him to feel both angry about working late and stressed out because he didn't believe his work was being recognized or compensated. The stress resulted in physical tension, which he felt all through his neck and back. In response to the feelings of anger, stress, and physical discomfort, Tom turned to a compensating habit. He would go to the office vending machine and purchase several candy bars that he would eat all at once, even though he was trying to lose weight.

Soon, eating the candy bars became more than just Tom's unhealthy habit; it became a new triggering event. Tom felt guilty about eating the candy bars because he was trying to lose weight. In turn, this made him feel ugly and fat. Feeling defeated, Tom's negative feelings led him to eat even more, which further discouraged him from restarting his healthy eating plan the next day.

Despite these self-perpetuating, unhealthy behaviors, Tom was able to break the chain by changing his thoughts about work. When he had to work late, he thought, "I have been given this work because they think I do a good job. But I cannot let my work get in the way of my health." With this new thought, Tom was able to change his feelings from negative ones of anger and stress to positive ones of pride in his work and a sense of control over his life. Feeling empowered to make the healthy changes he needed, Tom no longer needs sweets to get through the day.

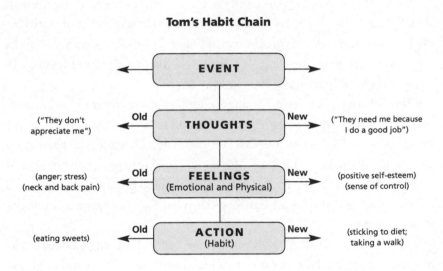

Tom's Habit Chain

Feelings

As you can see from Tom's habit chain, thoughts lead to feelings, and a change in thought can change feelings. In Tom's situation, his old thought led to feelings of anger and stress, while his new thought made him feel positive and more in control. Recognizing or acknowledging our feelings is not always easy, especially if we have never stopped to think about them before, and many of us don't. With old habits, in particular, we often move directly from a triggering event to the thought and then right to the action or habit we use as a coping mechanism, without stopping to observe the feelings we experience between the two. In many ways, we form our unhealthy habits in an effort to ignore or bypass our unwanted or uncomfortable feelings. Someone who is dealing with sadness and says, "I feel like eating a pint of ice cream," is sending out a powerful statement. Sugar and ice cream may indeed pacify uncomfortable feelings, but this person also may be trying to bury his or her sorrows.

According to Dr. Susan Jackubowitz, a psychotherapist who consults for the Active Wellness Program, the only way to stop an unhealthy habit is to "digest" or "own" the feelings that trigger and perpetuate the habit. This means you need to "feel" the feelings you are avoiding, not smother them with an unhealthy habit. When you allow yourself to feel those feelings—instead of jumping over them to a compensating habit—you may no longer need your old behavior. But first it is helpful to acknowledge and name the feelings you are experiencing, so you can feel in control and respond rather than react.

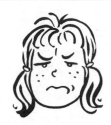

Mad

Sad

RECOGNIZING YOUR FEELINGS We all experience hundreds and hundreds of feelings of varying intensities. As you observe yourself in different situations, you will begin to recognize your unique way of feeling. Essentially, all feelings arise from four primal emotions: anger, grief, joy, and fear—or mad, sad, glad, and scared.

If you have trouble recognizing or acknowledging your feelings, you are not alone. Many of us hide our true feelings or ignore the messages they send us because we believe that showing our feelings is a sign of weakness, or the feelings themselves are unpleasant, so why pay attention to them.

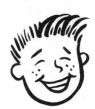

Glad

But feelings have a unique life force of their own. They are driven by powerful biochemical energies, and those energies need to be expressed and channeled in healthy and appropriate ways. Feelings, like food, need to be digested or they will cause physical and emotional "indigestion," which can cause us to feel emotionally "stuck" and unable to move toward our desired actions. How we feel emotionally can have a direct impact on how we feel physically, because the brain reacts to our mood and releases chemical messengers that affect our nervous and muscular system. This is one way the mind-body connection works. If we are afraid, we are familiar with the rapid

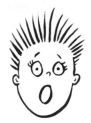

Scared

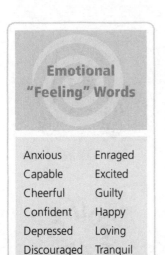

heartbeat, shallow breathing, cold sweats, and tight muscles that we experience. On the other hand, when we feel good, we are aware that we look better, are less tense, and cope more effectively with the situations life throws our way. By acknowledging your emotions, you can release the energy they carry and reduce the negative health effects you might otherwise experience if you either ignore your feelings or hold them in.

As you become familiar with recognizing your feelings, the best way to express them is to give yourself space to acknowledge them. Remember, feelings are never wrong. Not accepting your feelings—particularly the negative and uncomfortable ones—and keeping them locked inside ultimately affect both your health and your behavior.

Actions (Habits)

An action or habit is the last link in the event-thought-feeling-habit chain reaction. Often our unwanted habit is our way of coping with unwanted feelings that arise from our thoughts, which in turn began with the trigger that ignited the whole chain reaction. In some cases, a habit can actually arise as a coping mechanism to avoid positive feelings, such as fear of success. As in Tom's story, the initial action or habit (eating sweets to deal with anger) created a vicious cycle whereby new thoughts and feelings emerged that produced other unhealthy actions (giving up on his new healthy eating plan).

Four Coaching Tools for Change

Now that we have an understanding of how a habit is formed and how it can be broken, we can look at the different tools you can use to manage your triggers and create new habits.

Below is a selection of coaching tools you can use to change your habits. As you read through the different options, some will appeal to you more than others. I encourage you to work through each of the exercises here so that you have a good understanding of all the coaching tools at your disposal. Each tool will provide you with a slightly different strategy for breaking your old habit. As you proceed with your program, choose the strategies that make the most sense for you in the moment. As new situations arise, you

coach tip

Think about what actions you are taking that are serving you and how they make living a healthy lifestyle easier. What actions are you taking that are not serving you? Use the lessons in Step 1 to shift from your unwanted actions to useful actions. Although it takes conscious effort at first to change your actions, you don't have to take those actions that don't serve you.

will probably want to revisit this section to determine which coaching options will be most useful at different times.

1. Creating New Habits Using the Power of Thought and the Habit Chain

Many Active Wellness participants find it extremely helpful to fill out their own habit chain as practice in observing their self-talk. After reading each of the following instructions, take a moment to fill in your responses on the habit chain diagram provided on page 28 for your personal use:

Ⓐ *Identify the triggering event:* Think about a circumstance that happened that resulted in you taking an action you were not happy with. Write it on the fill-in rule beside "Event."

Ⓑ *Identify your thoughts or "self-talk":* For example, if your children are screaming, your thought or self-talk might be "I want to pull my hair out," or "I need a piece of chocolate to calm me down." Create your own self-talk statement and write it beside "Thoughts."

Ⓒ *Know your feelings:* It helps to understand how your thoughts affect how you feel. Often we use a habit to avoid feelings that arise from our thoughts. Try to remember how you felt both emotionally and physically as a result of the event. Describe these feelings on the appropriate line.

D *Identify your action (habit):* Look at the final action you took in reaction to your thoughts and feelings. Was it something you wanted to do? If it is difficult to pinpoint your triggering event, work backward. First, think about an action you took recently that you wish you could have prevented and write it on the line beside "Action (Habit)." Working backward is sometimes easier when you are reflecting on a past action.

E *Changing your thought:* Review your completed habit chain. Then try to come up with a new thought in response to one of your trigger events, one that is more positive and empowering or one that focuses on what you need to do for yourself. Notice if this thought leads to more positive feelings and then ask yourself, "Would I have taken the same action if I had changed my thoughts and had different feelings?"

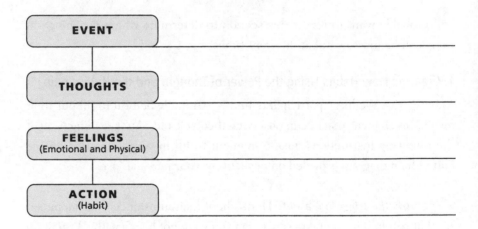

Your Habit Chain

2. Using Affirmations to Your Advantage

Another powerful tool you can use to deal with self-talk is affirmations. These are short, positive sayings that can encourage and empower you as you make positive changes in your life. They help counteract negative thoughts and feelings that might inhibit you from moving forward and reaching your goals. Below are examples of affirmations. Repeat them to yourself over and over during difficult times to help keep you on a positive track. Write them down on small index cards or Post-its and put them where you can see them every

Sometimes we have conversations with ourselves that we distinctly recognize, because they are discussions that we repeat continually. You may even sense a moment when you know a particular "self-talk" conversation is going to show up. When it is difficult not to listen to your "self-talk," try to change your perspective. Try looking for the humor in the situation and laugh at it. This can force you to develop a different viewpoint and often to achieve greater self-understanding. Know that you have the power to choose the perspective from which you view the conversations you have with yourself. When you can laugh at yourself, you may find yourself saying, "Here I go again, dallying in that old habit. Silly me. I am going to find a way out of this." Try on a new perspective in a familiar situation and see how it feels. What did you notice?

day: the bathroom mirror, the door to your bedroom, or the steering wheel of your car.

ACTIVE WELLNESS AFFIRMATIONS

I am doing the best I can.

I deserve time to focus on myself.

I am smart.

I am a good person.

You also can make personalized affirmations using the guidelines and space provided on page 30. You can even use a line from a favorite commercial, such as Nike's "Just Do It!" or a favorite inspirational quote.

When you start your day with a positive affirmation, you bring positive energy into the rest of your day and into all of your endeavors, including the process of changing unhealthy habits into healthy ones.

GUIDELINES FOR CREATING AFFIRMATIONS

Believe your affirmation to be true.

Use positive words and phrases, so your affirmation makes you feel good!

Use the present tense.

Use positive phrases that are in direct opposition to your old, negative self-talk.

If you're used to thinking, "I always fail," transform that into "I am a winner!"

Make your affirmation easy to remember.

My Personal Affirmations

_____

_____

_____

_____

_____

3. Managing Trigger Events with Substitution, Avoidance, and Elimination

When you can identify your trigger events, you can learn how to catch yourself before your habit affects how you feel and what you do. By learning to respond to an event, you can act proactively, rather than reactively, even though you may not be able to change or even be aware of all the triggers that occur in your life.

Below, the types of triggers are described and categorized as environmental, physiological, and emotional, to help you classify the types you experience. Once you have isolated and identified the unique triggering events in your life, you can use the tools of substitution, avoidance, and elimination for trigger management. As you read through the trigger descriptions, think about your own triggers and be prepared to fill in the exercises at the end of this section.

STEP 1: IDENTIFYING YOUR TRIGGER EVENTS

ENVIRONMENTAL TRIGGERS These triggers are anything you can see, hear, touch, smell, or taste.

Sound and touch: Loud noises or crashing sounds may trigger anxiety or anger, while touching something soft and warm may trigger feelings of comfort and security.

Smells: These can trigger you to eat when you really don't want to, or to eat the wrong things. When you walk into a movie theater and smell popcorn, you might feel pleasant anticipation of the movie that awaits you. Likewise, the sweet smells from a bakery can start your mouth watering as you walk by the shop's window.

Social events: Holidays or dining out with friends are also triggers. Indeed, just the thought of having to attend certain events or family get-togethers can set off an old behavior pattern or way of thinking. For many people, having food in front of them, particularly sweets, sets off most of the triggers that interfere with maintaining a healthy weight. The sight of them can be enough to push you off your wellness plan.

Caffeine: This substance can stimulate our appetite and give us temporary feelings of increased energy. A drop in energy often follows the peak

Case History: Environmental Triggers

When Jane first started her Active Wellness eating plan, she always had a difficult time refusing dessert when she was at a restaurant. This was particularly difficult at restaurants where she saw desserts displayed in a case or on a table before she was seated, an environmental trigger that sabotaged her eating plan. Compounding that, her boyfriend proved to be an additional environmental trigger. He always encouraged her to eat dessert, because he knew she really wanted it.

As hard as Jane tried to stick with one serving of dessert a day, restaurants remained a problem. For Jane, not eating something after she had dinner was too difficult, because she had been brought up to always have dessert after a meal. However, once she recognized her double triggers, she began to take actions to change her behavior. At first, she would order a dessert, but she would share it with others at the table. Soon, Jane stopped ordering dessert altogether and had fruit instead. She developed a new and pleasurable association with fruit by linking it to her memories of vacationing in the Caribbean.

of energy we feel when the effect of the caffeine dissipates. By eliminating or reducing caffeine, you may feel like you have more energy because your blood sugar is more even throughout the day.

People: People in your life can be environmental triggers and present interesting challenges to your healthy lifestyle. Without even knowing why, you may find that being around certain people encourages you to engage in old habits that you have been trying to avoid. Perhaps these people bring up uncomfortable feelings in you that make you want to reach for your old, compensating habit.

PHYSIOLOGICAL TRIGGERS Some of the most common physiological triggers include low blood sugar, fatigue, pain, and stress. They affect us physically, mentally, and emotionally, often making us feel out of control.

Low blood sugar: A drop in blood glucose levels can cause a person to feel dizzy, hungry, cranky, and tired, which may trigger a craving to eat anything in order to feel better. Most people with low blood sugar often reach for a candy bar or some type of sweet to "perk" them up again. While the re-

Case History: Physiological Triggers

Margaret's daily routine consisted of waking up at 5:30 A.M. to exercise for thirty minutes, commuting more than an hour to her office, working from 8:00 A.M. to 6:00 P.M., and then commuting back home. She often did not return home until 8:00 P.M. At that point, Margaret would always find herself craving sweets without knowing why. What she soon discovered was that fatigue was triggering food cravings.

Margaret's body naturally needed fuel to keep up its grueling schedule, and sugar is the fastest-acting form of fuel. But the effects of sugar don't last long, producing a self-perpetuating cycle of artificial "highs and lows" that encouraged Margaret's sugar cravings. The more highs and lows she experienced, the more fatigue she felt. Finally, Margaret arranged to do some stress-management techniques during her lunch break to help her relax and unwind during the day. At night, she consciously committed herself to getting more sleep. The better rested and more relaxed she became, the less she craved sugar.

fined carbohydrates, processed flour products, and sugar help us feel good and give us the short-term sugar high, unfortunately, in just a few hours the same sugar levels drop drastically, leaving us feeling fatigued, emotionally down, and craving another boost through carbohydrates or caffeine. People with diabetes are especially susceptible to the triggering effects of low blood sugar, as are those who skip meals as well as those who exercise strenuously on a regular basis but don't eat enough carbohydrates to sustain proper muscle functioning.

The need to feel calm: It is not unusual to crave foods made with refined flour (white flour) and sugar like bread, pasta, cakes, and cookies, because it helps to cause a calming chemical reaction in the brain known as the seratonin response, which helps us feel soothed. Therefore, when you are stressed or agitated, craving food to elevate your seratonin level is a natural way to feel better, especially if food was promoted as a source of comfort when you were a child.

Extreme fatigue: This is another physiological trigger, often sending messages to the body that it needs to eat to increase stamina. Some people are more susceptible than others to the various internal chemical reactions that influence stress, pain, anxiety, and hunger.

EMOTIONAL TRIGGERS Events or situations that make us feel we have lost control, succeeded, failed, increased responsibility, or been forced into making a major decision are some examples of emotionally charged circumstances that can trigger emotional feelings. When faced with such feelings, we often choose to avoid or "bury" them by procrastinating with an old habit, such as walking into the kitchen and eating whatever we see in the refrigerator or cupboard. Stress events that can lead to emotional triggers can include:

* new job
* change in routine
* argument
* project deadline
* waiting for a phone call you are expecting

Case History: Emotional Triggers

Anita, an Active Wellness participant who lived alone, felt loneliest in the evenings when she sat at home by herself. This was an especially difficult time for her because she had recently lost her husband, and they had always shared the hours after dinner together. Alone and lonely, Anita found it very hard not to snack after dinner: Food became the antidote for her loneliness. Once she understood that feeling lonely was a trigger for overeating, Anita was able to substitute new actions to alleviate her loneliness, ones that didn't involve food. She would call her sister or a friend whenever she felt particularly lonely, which helped her avoid overeating in the evening. Soon Anita was easily able to lose weight and achieve her Active Wellness primary goal.

STEP 2: WORKING WITH TRIGGERS: SUBSTITUTION, AVOIDANCE, AND ELIMINATION

SUBSTITUTION When you're "unlearning" old behaviors and habits, substituting something similar to, but healthier than, your old behavior is often the easiest solution. Your substitute trigger may take the form of a distraction, an action that helps you stop focusing on an unhealthy behavior and refocus on your health goals. For example, think about biting into a soft, chewy chocolate chip cookie that is still warm from the oven. The sweet taste and warm dough are soothing to your mouth and emotions. Now, stop thinking about the cookie and begin thinking about what it would be like to bite into a wedge of a fresh, tangy lemon. The tart taste of the lemon may even make you cringe. Did you make a face when you visualized this image? Did it take your mind off the cookie? Substitutions work well either when they distract you from your old habit or when they replace an unhealthy habit with a healthier alternative. Below are other examples of substitutions.

Trigger: Needing to order dessert in a restaurant
Substitution: Ordering fruit for dessert instead

Trigger: Taking coffee and snack breaks in the office coffee nook
Substitution: Drinking herbal iced or hot tea instead

Trigger: Taking a snack break at 3 P.M.
Substitution: Taking a walk around the block

Think about some of the triggers in your life that you would like to manage better by substituting healthier responses for them. Space has been provided in the Trigger Substitution box that follows. Write in three of the triggers that are most troublesome to you, using the examples above as a guide. Next, think of some behaviors that you can substitute for your old trigger behavior. Keep your substitution actions simple, direct, and easy to do so that they strengthen your commitment and motivation to change.

Your Trigger Substitution List

Trigger 1: _____

Substitution 1: _____

Trigger 2: _____

Substitution 2: _____

Trigger 3: _____

Substitution 3: _____

A very effective method for dealing with trigger substitutions is to prepare trigger cards you can carry with you. I call these Alternative Trigger Cards. To prepare your cards, write each trigger across the top of its own index card or piece of paper, and then beneath each write as many substitute behaviors as possible to counteract this trigger. I encourage you to create as many cards for as many triggers as you can and carry them with you wherever you go—in your briefcase, wallet, or purse.

Often we rely on our unhealthy habits for immediate gratification as a response to our feelings. Your best alternative behavior in the short term may be to quickly do something that is easy and accessible: calling a friend or family member; taking a walk or drive; or visiting the nearest mall to pamper yourself with a frivolous purchase.

You can review your alternative trigger cards on the spot and experiment with any of the substitute behaviors you have written down. To help you set up your card system, an example alternative trigger card, complete with substitute behaviors, appears below.

Alternative Trigger Card

Trigger: I eat whenever I am bored at work.

Alternative Options:
Write down a list of things I want to do for myself and do one.
Call or E-mail a friend for a quick hello.
Read a magazine article or look up a favorite topic on the Internet.
Eat something from my eating plan.

Identifying your triggers and devising strategies for managing them better are essential tasks for reinforcing and maintaining your new, healthy habits. With time, commitment, and simple repetition, your new behaviors and trigger-management techniques will become second nature. As you become aware of your triggers, it is helpful to think about why they appeared in your life, how they make you feel, and what they mean to you. Over time you'll be able to better manage your responses.

AVOIDANCE Avoidance is a legitimate strategy for managing triggers when you are just beginning to let go of old habits and adopt new ones. In the simplest of terms, you may need to stay away as much as possible from people, places, and things that trigger the impulse to return to unhealthy behaviors. This may include some friends and family members, at least on a temporary basis, as well as certain restaurants, pubs, social gatherings, family get-togethers, and even your favorite television show!

Review the triggers you listed on the previous page. Then, in the space provided below, write down those triggers you can reasonably avoid on a short-term basis while you begin the work on changing your unhealthy habits.

Triggers to Avoid

_____

_____

_____

_____

Testimonial

I never had to worry about my weight, but being downtown in New York City for 9/11 really threw me for a loop. Ever since that day, I have been using food as a tool to comfort myself. Before I knew it, I had gained twenty-five pounds in one year and I was having a difficult time controlling my blood sugars. I looked to Active Wellness for guidance, because I wanted to personalize a plan that would be designed to fit my needs.

When I first started the program, I realized which foods were my trigger foods, and I eliminated them from the house. Typically, when I would get home and feel stressed by family demands, I would grab a bag of chips; now I take five to ten minutes and work out on a machine I have at home. It is a great substitution because I control my stress, increase my energy for the evening, and burn calories to lose weight. Plus, I get to unwind from my workday with a few minutes to myself.

Sallyann, age thirty-four, just started program, lost five pounds in one month, blood sugar under better control

ELIMINATION When avoidance isn't possible, and substitution doesn't work, sometimes outright elimination is the only solution. Elimination refers to getting rid of something that has a negative effect on you and your wellness plan, and keeping it out of your life—for good. For example, to stay on your Active Wellness eating plan, you may need to eliminate certain foods and beverages from your kitchen shelves and your shopping list. To maintain your fitness plan, you may have to give up Wednesday night cocktails with the gang from work. To get enough sleep so that you can maintain your entire Active Wellness schedule, you may have to forego *The David Letterman Show*! In the space provided below, write down those triggers that you feel should be totally eliminated from your life.

Triggers to Eliminate

_____

_____

_____

_____

Identifying your triggers and devising strategies for managing them better are essential tasks for reinforcing and maintaining your new, healthy habits. With time, commitment, and simple repetition, your new behaviors and trigger-management techniques will become second nature. As you become aware of your triggers, it is helpful to think about why they appeared in your life, how they make you feel, and what they mean to you. Over time you'll be able to better manage your responses.

4. Managing Time as a Trigger

If we don't have enough time to make ourselves and our health a priority, the lack of time can become a trigger that induces stress and inhibits us from doing what we need to do to take care of ourselves. If you are under time pressure, you are more likely to seek out quick-fix alternatives that don't serve you, such as overeating food for comfort, or listening to television as an escape, reducing the time you have for fitness and effective stress-management techniques. Using some simple time-management tools, you can learn to carve out time for yourself and greatly reduce the likelihood that overplanning will get in the way of your Active Wellness routine.

Below is a Time Management Priority Chart to help you identify how to focus your time on tasks that are most important to you. Take a few minutes now to fill in what you would like to accomplish in the next day. Rank each activity according to its priority: A is most important, B is somewhat important, and C is not very important.

Time Management Priority Chart

Things to do today:	Priority Rating
	A = Most Important
	B = Somewhat Important
	C = Not Very Important
1.	
2.	
3.	
4.	
5.	
6.	
7.	

Review your completed list, and ask yourself the following:

1 Did you remember to include time for yourself? If not, write it in now. Time for yourself qualifies as an A task. In the long run, this will make you more productive in all aspects of your life, because you will be healthier, happier, and energized!

2 What if I can't complete all of these tasks today? If you think this is a possibility, cross out all the tasks that you have labeled as C, not very important. These tasks can wait until tomorrow.

3 Does your list seem manageable now? If not, cross out the B-level tasks. Now you can focus on what you really need to get done today—all of the A-level priorities.

DISTINGUISHING BETWEEN URGENT AND IMPORTANT ACTIVITIES

Prioritize your tasks by distinguishing between those tasks that are important and those tasks that are urgent. In a hectic workday, it is often difficult to decipher between the two, but learning to do so is part of time management.

> Important: Any task that matches your goals, values, and vision of what you want in your life. Urgent: Tasks immediately pressing upon you that must get accomplished right away. These tasks may not be important, but the urgency needed to accomplish them often puts them ahead of important "A" tasks on your to-do list. An urgent task may be taking a friend to the doctor, someone standing in your office asking a question, or a phone call you must take.

Often, important tasks such as purchasing healthful foods for your eating plan, setting aside time for fitness, and making time to schedule doctor appointments do not feel urgent, but if they are not included as "must do" A priorities on your to-do list, they will fall by the wayside because other urgent priorities get in the way.

Case History: Managing Time

Linda started the program because she wanted to lose weight. She is a nurse who works forty-six hours a week, she commutes three hours a day, and has a husband and two children waiting for her at home. Like many participants, Linda found it difficult to determine when she was going to make time for her Active Wellness Program. After trying different times, Linda decided to use her lunch hour. Once she identified an island of time for herself, she savored it every day. By finding "her" time, Linda was able to achieve and maintain her weight-loss goal and work at reducing her stress.

If not making time for yourself is a trigger, your task is to dedicate a specific time to accomplish your Active Wellness Program and do your best 95 percent of the time to not let anything interrupt this sacred time. The more consistent you are with setting time aside for yourself, the easier it will be for you to develop a regular routine that gets integrated into your life as a new healthy habit.

DESIGNING A REALISTIC DAILY SCHEDULE

Using your A and B priorities from your to-do list, make a schedule of your activities and commitments. You can use the Daily Activity Log below or your personal date book for this exercise.

Be aware of your personal "prime time"—the times of day when you do your best work. During these times, try to do the activities that require you to be the most alert. Don't forget to build in some free time for fun, relaxation, and exercise, as well as at least one hour for unexpected things. Although on paper it may look like you can get everything done, urgent things always come up during the day that can throw off even the best-laid plans. You want to leave time for the unexpected so that things don't become stressful in your day.

Making time to work on your program is critical to your success. Nothing can grow unless you devote attention to it. When all is said and done, remember to give yourself permission to do nothing at times.

Daily Activity Log

Time Allotted	Activity

REWARDING YOURSELF

Change is difficult, and you deserve a pat on the back for all of your efforts. In fact, sometimes I actually reach around my body and give myself a pat on the shoulder! Try it—it works. Acknowledging your good efforts and hard work is very important. Reinforcing your sense of accomplishment and self-worth strengthens your chances of reaching your long-term goals.

Try establishing a reward system for yourself. A reward should be something that feels special, that you don't always give yourself. Every time you practice your new healthy habit, for example, give yourself a dollar. At the end of every month, take the money you have saved and treat yourself to a gift—a new shirt, a bouquet of flowers, or a new CD. The reward is important because it is recognition of your efforts, by you. Change takes energy and focus, and often you are the only one who can relate to how much effort you are putting forth to reach your goals, so acknowledging your personal effort can be central to your success with your program. Using the Reward List below, take a moment now to jot down some of your short-terms goals and the rewards you can use to treat yourself when your goals have been accomplished. A list may seem simplistic, but it is actually a great tool when you're trying to make changes, because looking at your list forces you to stop and think before you act.

Reward List

Short-term Goals

_____

_____

_____

_____

Rewards

_____

_____

_____

_____

If you find yourself slipping at this or some future point in your wellness journey, take heart: Many have been there before you and gone on to become great successes. Changing lifelong behaviors that have stopped working for you is hard and courageous work. Give yourself credit for your hard work, and forgive yourself for any small setbacks.

Whenever you are learning anything new, you may have to take a few steps backward to reassess your progress and your techniques before you can move more confidently forward to success. Minor failures are an integral part of the learning process. The important thing is to avoid getting stuck for too long when you have a slip or two. Missteps and stumbles are important junctures in your program, and how quickly you handle them may make the difference between long-term success or self-defeat, lifelong wellness or chronic bad health.

Being Human Means Making Mistakes

In terms of taking control of our health, each of us has a personal "Waterloo," a breaking point or testing point at which we feel so defeated and powerless that we are tempted to throw in the towel completely. One moment we are strolling confidently along our wellness path; the next moment we stumble and find ourselves falling into a deep hole that seems to offer no way out.

As you make healthy changes in your life, remember to go easy on yourself. Abandoning old, ingrained habits that have served you well for years is hard work. Thinking that you are not "okay" if you don't succeed immediately, or do something perfectly, is wrong—if not downright counterproductive. Remember, success is when you continue to try, and failure is when you give up.

I tell all my Active Wellness clients that they are expected to make mistakes. Great learning comes from making mistakes. And if you are constantly worried about doing something wrong, more of your energy is devoted to worrying than it is to learning new information and making healthy changes. Often, what we want comes to us more easily when we stop worrying about it.

Being human means making mistakes and not being perfect. A minor setback in your eating plan may occur, such as ordering a rich and fattening dessert in a restaurant or devouring the chips and nuts at the bar while you wait for a table. Such an occurrence can begin a relentless barrage of negative self-talk where you set yourself up as a "failure." You may be tempted to give up on your wellness plan entirely, perhaps believing yourself incapable of truly eating healthfully and losing weight. Instead, you need to gently encourage yourself with positive thoughts and affirmations.

Turn setbacks into new opportunities. When you "feel" stuck, this can be an important clue about a major roadblock you may have to face and understand in order to move forward. By overcoming these roadblocks you will feel stronger and more confident. When you can stop and feel whole, just as you are, with your imperfections and limitations, you can be at peace with yourself and begin the real work of making changes that last a lifetime. Life is not meant to be a trap where we live constantly on guard. We are meant to enjoy life and the day-to-day process of learning to be healthy human beings. As you change your thoughts and feelings and uncover the unconscious forces that get in the way of your conscious objectives, you will begin to achieve some of your goals. You'll begin to accept more and more who you are and where you are. Only you can decide what's important for you and how you're going to get it. And if that sometimes means you have to toot your own horn and be selfish about your needs, so be it!

Change Can Be Scary . . .

Remember that any effort to improve yourself is worthwhile. If you are having trouble moving forward and taking those first steps toward change, ask yourself several questions:

> If I take action, what is the best thing that can happen because of my efforts?
>
> If I take action, what is the worst thing that can happen because of my efforts?
>
> If I don't take action, what am I getting from holding on to my old behavior?

You may find that the worst thing that can happen isn't so bad and that the chance you take toward healthy change is more than worth the risk, espe-

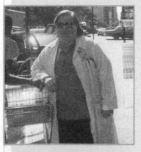

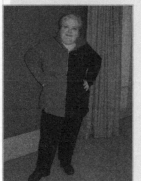

I knew I needed to do something to help myself. I wasn't happy the way I was—overweight and unhealthy with uncontrolled blood pressure. I always knew I wasn't cut out to be on a diet—I am not good at being told what to do. I needed something that was going to help me mentally take control of my habits and behaviors. Then I was introduced to Active Wellness, which appealed to me because its realistic and flexible strategies gave me personal choice. One of the first things I learned was how to combat my triggers—this is what really helped me make changes. I was afraid of failing at first. But Active Wellness gave me the tools and knowledge to make healthier changes. I learned how to be creative with my food choices. Now I pay attention to the food I am eating, the flavor, the variety, and the presentation. I enjoy my food more and I eat less.

With Active Wellness, it was about taking care of yourself in a healthy way. I didn't feel like I had to follow a strict program and if I went off, it was all over. With Active Wellness, once in a while I am not as diligent, but since you learn what you need to know, you have the confidence that you can start right up again with your program. I know this will be for a lifetime because it is livable. It is a way of life, not a diet. My self-esteem has gone up so much and I feel so good that it is affecting my spirit and the rest of my life.

Elaine, age fifty, lost 50 pounds and cut blood pressure medication in half, dropped 5 sizes in clothing

cially when the benefits you reap are wellness and weight management for a lifetime.

You now have empowering techniques for managing slips and temporary roadblocks. By remaining open about changing your old beliefs and devising healthy substitutions for negative thoughts and actions, you can transform bad habits into healthy actions! You are ready to start planning your Active Wellness Program. The next step is to create your personal eating plan.

Main Points to Forming New Healthy Habits and Conquering Triggers That Sabotage Your Success

✔ The Active Wellness coaching tools provide you with strategies to change unwanted, unhealthy habits into healthy, satisfying behaviors.

✔ You first need to be aware of your bad habits in order to change them.

✔ Identifying your triggers can help you understand situations or events that stimulate your old habits and unwanted behaviors. Triggers can include thoughts, things in your environment, emotions, physiological responses, foods, and lack of time.

✔ New habits can be created by changing your perception and thoughts or physically changing your action.

✔ It takes focus and energy to make changes. It is important to acknowledge and reward yourself for your efforts.

Getting Started with Your Personal Eating Plan: Rethinking Food, Fat, and Calories

YOUR EATING PLAN is the cornerstone of your Active Wellness Program. Therefore, designing and following a personalized eating plan to fit your specific nutritional needs and wellness requirements is one of the most important factors in achieving your goals. Optimal nutrition strengthens and nourishes you physically, mentally, and emotionally. It prepares you to practice and enjoy the other components of the program—physical exercise, stress management, and maintaining your Active Wellness lifestyle.

Whatever your long-term and short-term goals are, this chapter will show you the types, combinations, and amounts of food you need to eat every day in order to achieve any one of a variety of weight-management and wellness goals.

Before you can begin to create your personalized eating plan, it is important to reframe your notion of what good nutrition is and isn't.

Myth vs. Fact

Myth: There is a special combination of foods that will help you lose weight.

Fact: Certain types of foods do not help you lose weight. Weight loss occurs when the amount of energy (calories) you take into your body through food exceeds the amount of energy you expend through your body's metabolism (functioning) and your exercise (activity). If you eat more calories than your body can convert into healthy energy, or you eat too many of the wrong kinds of calories, the excess energy left over in your body turns into fat and re-mains in your body as "storage fuel."

Storing fat as fuel for some future emergency is a survival mechanism left over from our ancient ancestors who faced famine on a regular basis and needed to utilize their bodies' reserves of fat simply to live. The average American rarely faces famine yet regularly packs away more storage fat than our ancestors ever dreamed of having. Fat is the culprit in obesity as well as a contributing factor to heart disease, cancer, and diabetes.

Myth: Carbohydrates make you gain weight and are unhealthy.

Fact: There are many popular fad diets that ask you to eliminate or reduce carbohydrates—grains, starches, fruits, and vegetables—and consume mostly proteins. First, carbohydrates don't make you fat. Fat is the result of eating more food than your body needs, and this can happen from any type of food, carbohydrate, fat, or protein. Eliminating carbohydrates from your diet is not healthy for your body. Your brain, muscles, and nervous system run on car-bohydrates. When your body is short on carbohydrates it breaks down your muscles to create carbohydrates to use as fuel. When you reduce carbohy-drates in your diet, your body is missing out on the protective benefits of the nutrients found in low-fat sources or carbohydrates. Therefore, it is much healthier to make sure you are eating carbohydrates every day.

Myth: Losing weight should happen quickly.

Fact: Research indicates that a weight loss of a half pound to two pounds a week is the best way to lose weight and keep it off. When you lose weight at a slow and steady pace you are losing body fat. When you lose weight quickly, chances are that the weight loss you are reading on the scale is mostly water loss with some loss of muscle and little, if any, fat loss.

Water loss occurs because your system is breaking down glycogen, the storage fuel from glucose you have in your liver. This releases water, and the increased intake of protein causes your body to use water to flush out the ketones or excess waste products from protein. When your body is in ketosis, because it doesn't have enough carbohydrates to use as fuel, the acidity in your blood increases and there is a change in the way some of your organs function, particularly your kidneys.

A loss of water weight does not improve your health status. The weight loss you want is fat loss, because it is the percentage of fat on your body that leads to health risks. High-protein diets are inherently high in animal fat, which is the "bad" fat that can increase our risk for disease. The American Heart Association, the American Diabetes Association, and the National Cancer Institute all concur that a balanced, low-fat diet is the healthiest diet you can eat.

Myth: In order to lose weight, you are supposed to be hungry.
Fact: If you are eating healthy foods in a balance that works with your body, you should not feel hungry. The correct foods in the correct proportions is the key to feeling satisfied with a healthy eating plan. When you eat correctly, you do not have cravings, you increase your energy, and you do not slow down your metabolism. Your body is a fine-tuned machine: When you supply it with the foods it needs, it runs fine; when you cut back on food, your metabolism can slow down, you will not lose weight, your body conserves what energy it has, and it doesn't function as well as if it were getting the right nutrients in the right amounts. If your metabolism is sluggish, it can affect how you feel and how energetically and effectively you perform your daily tasks.

Myth: All fats are bad.
Fact: Despite diets that promote the consumption of any and all fats as the way to lose weight, there are "good"/healthy and "bad"/unhealthy fats. Healthy fats are plant-based, including those derived from and found in

seeds, nuts, avocados, and olives. These good fats are liquid at room temperature, and are actually beneficial to your body's functioning.

"Bad" fats can cause high cholesterol levels, fatty plaque deposits in arteries, and cardiovascular disease. In general, these saturated fats are solid at room temperature and include animal fats, full-fat dairy products, and meats, as well as palm kernel oil, butter, and coconut oil. Another kind of fat, hydrogenated fat, is made from oils but is hardened through the addition of hydrogen. Margarine is a hydrogenated fat. Hydrogenated (and partially hydrogenated) fats are just as bad for you as saturated fats, if not worse, because when heated they produce trans-fatty acids, which have been linked to damage that may contribute to cancer, heart disease, and premature aging.

Myth: High insulin levels make you gain weight.
Fact: Insulin is the hormone that is responsible for transporting both glucose (blood sugars) and fats (triglycerides) to the cells after a meal. The presence of insulin does not mean you will gain weight. In fact, a healthy body functions by having insulin pull sugars and fats into your cells for use as fuel. The amount of nutrients that will be stored by your body will depend on whether you have eaten more food than your body needs. When you eat more than you expend, then insulin does serve to deposit fat and you will gain weight. It is overeating and not insulin that makes you gain weight.

Myth: Doctors know nutrition and understand how to give you eating recommendations.
Fact: Most doctors never went to school for nutrition. While doctors are well versed on how to prescribe diets, they have not been taught how to translate your diet needs into the foods you eat everyday. Unfortunately, many medical-school curriculums left out nutrition as a course of study. There is currently a shift to more nutrition education for doctors, but this is basic nutrition covered in one course. Registered Dietitians are nutrition professionals. In order to become a Registered Dietitian, you must complete at least two to three years of study and a minimum of 900 hours in an internship applying your nutrition knowledge to actual situations that cover diabetes, heart disease, digestion, healthy eating, physical disability, aging, and any other factor that contributes to a variation in nutritional requirements.

Creating Your Personal Plan

Now that we've dispelled some myths, let's get started in creating your healthy-eating program.

There are six nutrient categories that are considered essential to life:

Water	Proteins
Vitamins	Carbohydrates
Minerals	Fats

Of these six nutrients, *only* proteins, carbohydrates, and fats can be transformed into fuel for your body, which is measured in calories. In addition to providing you with energy, each of these nutrients plays its own distinct role in your body. Proteins build and repair muscles, bones, tissues, and skin. Carbohydrates turn into pure fuel to run the body. Fats are converted into either stored or excess fuel; in the case of essential fatty acids, these "good" fats help protect the body by promoting immune function, rebuilding cell membranes, and lowering blood levels of total cholesterol.

Your Active Wellness Program includes lean proteins, healthy carbohydrates, and "good" fats in proportions that are correct to meet your needs. You *will not* have to give up any one nutrient, since they are all important. The Active Wellness Program is designed to be practical and flexible. It gives you an opportunity to be creative with your food choices, so that no matter where you are, you can find food that fits into your program. With your Active Wellness eating plan, you will learn strategies so you can enjoy your meals, avoid cravings, and not overeat.

Your Nutrient Requirements—The First Step in Creating Your Eating Plan

Your body's energy requirements are unique to you. They depend on many factors, including your height, weight, age, gender, activity level, and general health. Therefore, the number of calories you need to consume as energy every day to feel good and perform well is also unique to you.

The best combination of foods for you to eat to maintain or lose weight will depend on your health needs. The first step in creating such an eating plan is determining how much energy your body needs every day. Weight loss will occur when you take in less energy than you expend. This creates a deficit of energy that leads to a depletion of fat storage.

Setting Realistic Weight-Loss Goals

Knowing your best weight level and choosing a reasonable weight-loss goal are the first requirements for setting up a customized eating plan. To help you determine your weight range, refer to the Weight for Height charts that appear on the next few pages.

If you generally have not been overweight during the past ten years but weight gain has become a fairly recent problem, use the Weight for Height Chart I. According to this chart, a reasonable weight range for a 5-foot, 8-inch woman is 130 to 150 pounds. If you have been very heavy or overweight for most of your life, use the Weight for Height Chart II. According to this chart, a reasonable weight range for a 5-foot, 8-inch woman is 175 to 187 pounds.

If the weight ranges from either chart seem too high or too low for you, ask yourself the following questions:

1 Have I always been on the thin or heavy side? If you have always been on the thin side or are small-boned, choose the lower end of the weight range for your height (the bottom number + 5 to 10 pounds). If you are

Don't weigh yourself every day! Weight fluctuates from day to day, depending on a variety of factors. Seeing a gain of 2 or 3 pounds when you've been sticking to your eating plan can be discouraging. If you feel you *must* weigh yourself, do it once every two weeks or once a month. Your progress will be abundantly clear, and your commitment to your program will be renewed.

large-boned or on the heavy side, choose the higher end of the weight range.

2 Have I been this weight during the last ten years and have I been able to maintain it, plus or minus 2 pounds? If the weight you choose for yourself is one you have maintained for a year or more sometime during the last ten years, it is probably a reasonable goal.

Weight for Height Chart I*

Use this chart if you are at a good weight or if you have put on weight during the last ten years.

Women		Men	
Height	**Weight**	**Height**	**Weight**
5 ft.	90–110	5 ft.	96–116
5 ft. 1 in.	95–115	5 ft. 1 in.	102–122
5 ft. 2 in.	100–120	5 ft. 2 in.	108–128
5 ft. 3 in.	105–125	5 ft. 3 in.	114–134
5 ft. 4 in.	110–130	5 ft. 4 in.	120–140
5 ft. 5 in.	115–135	5 ft. 5 in.	126–146
5 ft. 6 in.	120–140	5 ft. 6 in.	132–152
5 ft. 7 in.	125–145	5 ft. 7 in.	138–158
5 ft. 8 in.	130–150	5 ft. 8 in.	144–164
5 ft. 9 in.	135–155	5 ft. 9 in.	150–170
5 ft. 10 in.	140–160	5 ft. 10 in.	156–176
5 ft. 11 in.	145–165	5 ft. 11 in.	162–182
6 ft.	150–170	6 ft.	168–188
6 ft. 1 in.	155–175	6 ft. 1 in.	174–194
6 ft. 2 in.	160–180	6 ft. 2 in.	180–200
6 ft. 3 in.	165–185	6 ft. 3 in.	186–206
6 ft. 4 in.	170–190	6 ft. 4 in.	192–212

*Based on the Hamwai Method for Determining Ideal Body Weight, a standard equation used to estimate weight for height.

Weight for Height Chart II*

Use this chart to determine your weight if you have been overweight or very heavy for most of your life.

Women		Men	
Height	**Weight**	**Height**	**Weight**
5 ft.	125–128	5 ft.	133–145
5 ft. 1 in.	131–144	5 ft. 1 in.	140–152
5 ft. 2 in.	138–150	5 ft. 2 in.	148–160
5 ft. 3 in.	144–156	5 ft. 3 in.	155–168
5 ft. 4 in.	150–162	5 ft. 4 in.	162–175
5 ft. 5 in.	156–168	5 ft. 5 in.	170–182
5 ft. 6 in.	163–175	5 ft. 6 in.	178–190
5 ft. 7 in.	169–181	5 ft. 7 in.	185–197
5 ft. 8 in.	175–187	5 ft. 8 in.	193–205
5 ft. 9 in.	181–193	5 ft. 9 in.	200–212
5 ft. 10 in.	188–200	5 ft. 10 in.	208–220
5 ft. 11 in.	194–206	5 ft. 11 in.	215–227
6 ft.	200–212	6 ft.	223–235
6 ft. 1 in.	206–218	6 ft. 1 in.	230–242
6 ft. 2 in.	212–224	6 ft. 2 in.	238–250
6 ft. 3 in.	219–231	6 ft. 3 in.	245–269
6 ft. 4 in.	225–237	6 ft. 4 in.	253–265

*Based on the Hamwai Method for Determining Ideal Body Weight, a standard equation used to estimate weight for height.

Record Your Weight Goal Here:_____

Now that you have established a reasonable weight goal for yourself, you are ready to choose your daily calorie level, one that promotes weight loss or maintains your current weight and also targets specific health conditions.

How Much Energy Does Your Body Need?

Energy, in the form of food calories, is needed for digestion, physical activity, and healing the body. The amount of calories that your body requires varies with age, gender, and height. To determine how much energy your body needs, you should know about how many calories your body burns as fuel on a daily basis. The Daily Calorie Intake charts on the following pages will help you determine what your ideal daily calorie/energy intake should be, whether for weight loss or weight maintenance, based on your height.

If you want to lose weight, find your height and the corresponding daily calorie level in the "Weight Loss" column. If you want to maintain your current weight, find your height in the first column and the corresponding maximum daily calorie level in the "Weight Maintenance" column.

Women's Daily Calorie (Energy) Intake Chart for Weight Loss and Weight Maintenance

Height	Maximum Calorie (Energy) Intake for Weight Loss	Maximum Calorie (Energy) Intake for Weight Maintenance*
5 ft.	1,200	1,400
5 ft. 1 in.	1,200	1,400
5 ft. 2 in.	1,300	1,500
5 ft. 3 in.	1,300	1,500
5 ft. 4 in.	1,400	1,600
5 ft. 5 in.	1,500	1,700
5 ft. 6 in.	1,500	1,700
5 ft. 7 in.	1,600	1,800
5 ft. 8 in.	1,600	1,800
5 ft. 9 in.	1,700	1,900
5 ft. 10 in.	1,800	2,000
5 ft. 11 in.	1,800	2,000
6 ft.	1,900	2,100
6 ft. 1 in.	1,900	2,100
6 ft. 2 in.	2,000	2,200
6 ft. 3 in.	2,000	2,200
6 ft. 4 in.	2,100	2,300

*Calorie levels for weight maintenance take into consideration that you have incorporated an exercise plan into your routine three or four times a week, for a minimum of 30 minutes per session. If you do not meet this minimum level of exercise, follow the calorie level indicated for weight loss.

Men's Daily Calorie (Energy) Intake Chart for Weight Loss and Weight Maintenance

Height	Maximum Calorie (Energy) Intake for Weight Loss	Maximum Calorie (Energy) Intake for Weight Maintenance*
5 ft.	1,200	1,400
5 ft. 1 in.	1,300	1,500
5 ft. 2 in.	1,300	1,500
5 ft. 3 in.	1,400	1,600
5 ft. 4 in.	1,500	1,700
5 ft. 5 in.	1,500	1,700
5 ft. 6 in.	1,600	1,800
5 ft. 7 in.	1,700	1,900
5 ft. 8 in.	1,700	1,900
5 ft. 9 in.	1,800	2,000
5 ft. 10 in.	1,900	2,100
5 ft. 11 in.	1,900	2,100
6 ft.	2,000	2,200
6 ft. 1 in.	2,000	2,200
6 ft. 2 in.	2,200	2,400
6 ft. 3 in.	2,200	2,400
6 ft. 4 in.	2,400	2,600

*Calorie levels for weight maintenance take into consideration that you have incorporated an exercise plan into your routine three or four times a week, for a minimum of 30 minutes per session. If you do not meet this minimum level of exercise, follow the calorie level indicated for weight loss.

Record Your Maximum Daily Caloric Level Here:_____

Most people want to lose weight and are reasonable about setting a healthy weight goal but not realistic about the time frame in which they can lose their excess weight. At first, everyone looks for "the quick fix"—10 pounds in one to two weeks. But it soon becomes apparent that a steady weight-loss goal of an average of 1 to 2 pounds per week is a comfortable, effective rate for long-lasting results. When you lose weight at a slow and

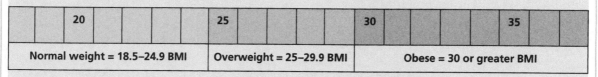

Body Mass Index (BMI)

This measure is a height-to-weight comparison that indicates excess body fat. If your BMI is over 25, you are at greater risk for diseases associated with excess weight. You can figure out your score with the following equation:

BODY MASS INDEX SCORE = 703 × your weight in pounds ÷ (your height in inches × your height in inches)

	20				25				30				35		
Normal weight = 18.5–24.9 BMI					Overweight = 25–29.9 BMI				Obese = 30 or greater BMI						

Source: National Institutes of Health, 1998

steady pace you are more likely to keep it off, because you have taken the time to integrate new healthy habits into your routine and find healthy foods you enjoy eating.

One pound of weight is equal to 3,500 calories. Even if you lower your food intake by 500 calories a day, which is what many of you who want to lose weight will be doing on your plan, it will take seven days to lose 1 pound (7 × 500 calories = 3,500 calories [1 lb]). If you exercise and burn even more energy (calories), you can lose 1 to 2 pounds on average per week. If you lose more weight at first, it is because you have lost some water weight. This will make you feel good, but it is not fat weight, so if you stop right away on your plan, you are bound to put this weight right back on.

Some weeks you may notice larger drops in weight than others, but keep in mind that you can be losing weight and not detect it on the scale for several weeks. Be patient, because by following your eating and exercising plans, your excess weight will come off.

Translating Your Calorie Level into Foods You'll Enjoy Eating

Now that you've identified your weight goal and determined your daily calorie level, you can apply your calorie level to specific food groups to design the framework of your eating plan.

You need to adjust your calorie level if you are forty years or older, because your metabolism slows down from a loss of muscle mass. Here's how to do it:

If you are in your forties: Deduct ½ percent per year from your total calories for every year between forty and fifty. So, if you are forty-three, that would mean a 1½ percent deduction in calories from the number you located on the chart.

If you are fifty-one years of age or older: Your calorie level drops by 1 percent per year, or 10 percent per decade. Therefore, if you are in this age group, you should adjust your caloric requirement by 5 percent to account for years forty to fifty, plus 1 percent for your fifty-first year, for a total decrease of 6 percent from the caloric total you estimated on the chart. The equations below can help you:

If you are between the ages of forty and fifty:
(Chosen calorie level) × [100 − (.005 × # of years in your forties) = new calorie level

If you are fifty-one years of age or older:
(Chosen calorie level) × [100 − (.5 (to account for your forties) + (.01 × # of years past fifty)] = new calorie level

Never go below 1,200 calories per day, even if your equation indicates a lower caloric number.

THE FOOD GROUPS

Your Active Wellness plan is a nutritionally balanced breakdown of a variety of low-fat foods that will promote good health. The food groups, plus alcohol and water, each designated by its own symbol, include:

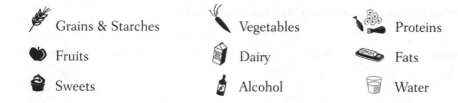

Grains & Starches   Vegetables   Proteins

Fruits   Dairy   Fats

Sweets   Alcohol   Water

The food groups and their symbols are used in your Active Wellness healthy-eating plan to identify categories of foods and servings. The amount of servings you have on your plan is defined by the caloric level you determined earlier in this step.

As you look at the Active Wellness Basic Eating Plan for Good Health chart, pictured on the next page, you will see that the symbols correspond to seven food groups plus alcohol and water. These are the food groups that are included in your plan. The Basic Eating Plan for Good Health is based on a balanced daily intake, with 50 percent carbohydrate, 25 percent protein, and 25 percent fat (primarily from unsaturated plant fats).

Refer to this same chart to locate the caloric level that corresponds to what you've chosen for yourself. In the same row as your caloric level, you will find the number of servings from each food group that you may eat every day to meet your nutritional needs. Feel free to circle this row to make it easy to identify.

For example, if you have chosen a calorie level of 1,600, you may eat the following each day:

6 servings of Grains/Starches
4 servings of Vegetables
6 servings of Protein
3 servings of Fruit
2 servings of Dairy
5 servings of Fat
1 serving of Sweets
1 optional serving of Alcohol

Don't worry about calculating how much food belongs in a serving. All of this is done for you later in this chapter in the Active Wellness Guide to

Active Wellness Basic Eating Plan for Good Health

Calorie Level	Grains/ Starches	Veggie	Protein	Fruit	Dairy	Fat	Sweets	Alcohol
1,200	3	3+	4	2	2	4	1	1
1,300	4	3+	5	2	2	4	1	1
1,400	4	4+	5	3	2	4	1	1
1,500	5	4+	6	2	3	4	1	1
1,600	6	4+	6	3	2	5	1	1
1,700	6	5+	6	3	2	6	1	1
1,800	7	4+	7	3	2	6	1	1
1,900	7	4+	8	3	3	6	1	1
2,000	8	4+	8	3	3	6	1	1
2,100	8	4+	8	3	3	7	1	1
2,200	9	4+	9	3	3	7	1	1
2,300	9	5+	9	3	3	8	1	1
2,400	10	5+	10	4	3	8	1	1
2,500	11	5+	10	4	3	9	1	1
2,600	11	6+	11	4	3	9	1	1

For all calorie levels, drink a minimum of 8 glasses of water a day.

Foods and Serving Sizes (see p. 84), which lists a variety of foods from each food group, together with their appropriate serving sizes.

For the first week or two, until you feel confident about choosing foods and designing meal plans, you may want to follow the Starter Plan at the end of this chapter. It provides a menu of foods and servings that you can use as a guide while you are getting established in your new eating routine. I encourage you to use the Starter Plan and to expand on the food choices listed in the plan by including other foods from each of the food groups. Always try to aim for a variety of tastes, textures, and colors in your meals, which will help keep your food interesting and appetizing.

If you have special health concerns, refer to the eating plans in the appendix that are designed specifically for the following concerns:

* Osteoporosis Prevention and Menopause
* Heart Disease, Stroke, Elevated Cholesterol, and High Blood Pressure
* Type 1 Insulin-Dependent and Type 2 Non–Insulin Dependent Diabetes, Insulin Resistance, Carbohydrate Cravings, and Hypoglycemia
* Individuals with a Personal or Family History of Cancer

In the appendix you can also find Special Dietary Guidelines that adjust your energy needs for high-intensity athletics, pregnancy, and breast-feeding. There is also a list of special eating considerations if you have conditions such as gout or lactose intolerance that affect the types of foods you should eat. Please refer to page 219 in the appendix for the Special Dietary Guidelines.

Using Your Plan Every Day

Now that you've laid the groundwork for designing a customized eating plan that's unique to your needs, let's begin putting it all together so that you can live with it every day. You won't be counting calories in the foods you eat on this plan. Instead, you'll be keeping track of the types and amounts of foods you eat to ensure that you are getting a good balance of the right nutrients every day.

Making smart food choices—not counting calories—is the key to eating healthfully, getting optimal nutrition, and preventing disease. Counting calories has an inherent danger because it may inadvertently encourage cheating: Those 260 calories you allotted for breakfast can include a banana and a bowl of cereal with low-fat milk—or they can be used to quickly eat a chocolate bar.

*
coach
tip

You can lose an average of two pounds a week safely and be well on the way to a leaner and healthier you.

Getting Started: Using Your Daily Allowance Card— "Your Daily Bank Account of Food"

You will use the Daily Allowance Card on page 62 to track your eating. There is a Daily Allowance Card in the appendix (on page 239), from which you can make copies to track your eating.

This is a learning tool that will help you understand how much food you can eat to meet your body's needs. It lists the food groups that comprise your

Daily Allowance Card

	No.	□ Daily Vitamins and Supplements
Water	8	
Grains & Starches	6	
Veggie	4+	
Protein	6	
Fruits	3	
Dairy	2	
Fats	5	
Sweets	1	
Alcohol	1	

plan and the distinctive symbols for each of the food groups. Each symbol on the card represents one serving. In the column next to the food group name, fill in the number of daily servings your eating plan allows.

Once you have entered the serving numbers on your Daily Allowance Card, you are ready to begin recording the foods you eat. To keep track of the number of servings you are eating in each food group, cross off the corresponding servings on your Daily Allowance Card. For foods not listed, either use the serving sizes on the package, or estimate a serving based on the information given for similar foods in your Active Wellness Guide to Foods and Serving Sizes, listed at the back of this step.

At the end of the day, you can review your eating patterns and see where you may have "overspent" your food budget or scrimped on nutrition. Think of your daily allotment of foods as your "nutrition bank account"—the card helps you to keep track of how you "spend" your food portions. It is up to you to decide when you would like to eat them.

At a minimum, the Daily Allowance Cards should be used for the first two weeks that you are on the Active Wellness eating plan. From the time you wake up until the time you go to bed, check off everything you eat on your card. If you "underspend" and have servings left over at the end of the day, don't worry. It is more important to be concerned if you find yourself "overspending" by eating more food than your daily allowance. If this is the case, just make a note of it and start anew the next day. *Take your new eating plan one day at a time.* Don't focus on how much weight you're losing, but on how good you're feeling!

Many of my clients begin tracking the foods they are eating by writing them down first in a food diary, which looks like the diagram below, and then translating the food into servings on their Daily Allowance Card. If you would like to use a food diary to record the foods you are eating, there are templates in the appendix for you to use.

Keep your Daily Allowance Card and Food Diary on your refrigerator or with your appointment calendar to help you remember to fill them out.

Date:_____   Eating Plan Weekly Goal:_____

Daily Food Diary

Time of Day	Food Eaten	Amount	Were you hungry before you ate? Yes / No

Daily Fitness and Stress Management Diary

Time of Day	Activity	Level of Intensity	Did You Meet Your Goal?

---

coach tip

Tracking your portions helps you to see where you are overspending on your daily bank account of food. It is easy to overeat on certain foods, particularly fats, because they contain more than twice the energy (9 calories per gram) than either protein (4 calories per gram) or carbohydrate (4 calories per gram). So, watch those fats and use them wisely!

Giving You Flexibility

Rules on Trading Servings You Don't Use or Counting Items that Are Not Low Fat

It is always better to acknowledge what you are eating, even if you think you were not following the plan exactly right. So, please use the following guidelines when you need more flexibility:

1. **You can trade your Sweet and Alcohol serving:** If you don't spend your Sweet or Alcohol, they can be traded for anything on your Daily Allowance Card, and you can trade one for the other, if necessary—i.e., if you don't have your Alcohol one day, you can trade the Alcohol for a serving of any other food or a sweet. But you can't save your alcohol up to use more than one serving a day, because that is unhealthy for your body.

2. **When a food is not low fat:** For any food that *is not* low fat (3 grams of fat or less/serving) or light—having 4 grams of fat (in the case of many light cheeses), you need to *add a Fat per serving* for each of these foods. For example, there are typically two servings of regular full-fat cheese on a slice of pizza. The cheese would count as 2 Dairy (for the cheese) and 2 Fats, one for each serving of cheese, since the cheese was not low fat.

3. **On the odd occasion you may indulge in a food that is deep fried:** If this is the case, *add 2 Fats per serving* for whatever food item it is. For French fries, for example, approximately ten are a serving. Since potato is a starch, that means you would have 1 Starch and 2 Fats. *You will soon see that your fat allowance can go quickly if you do not focus on mainly eating a low-fat diet.*

4. **Try not to trade other food portions you don't eat:** Do notice if you are continually missing a food group on your Daily Allowance Card and make a goal that will help you incorporate that food group into your eating plan.

5. **If you eat more than your allotted servings of Dairy:** Count additional Dairy as Protein, if you tend to eat more than your daily allowance. You can also trade your servings for Alcohol or a Sweet to increase your Dairy servings.

coach tip

The Facts You Need to Know About Healthy Eating

The Active Wellness Basic Food and Nutrition Guidelines

✳ *Eat low-fat foods as the mainstay of your daily eating plan.* Purchase individual food items that have 3 grams or less of total fat per serving or prepared meals that have 30 percent or less of total calories from fat. *Soy products and fish high in omega-3 fatty acids are exceptions to this guideline.*

All packaged foods are marked with nutrition facts labels like the one on the right. A good rule of thumb to follow when choosing low-fat foods is to check the nutrition label on the packages. By following this guideline you will also be limiting your saturated fat intake, since most low-fat foods are also low in saturated fat. Saturated fat can contribute to elevated cholesterol.

Nutrition Facts		
Serving Size 1 cup (228g)		
Servings Per Container 2		
Calories 80		
Calories from Fat 0g		
Amount Per Serving		**% Daily Value***
Total Fat 0		**0%**
Saturated Fat 0g		0%
Cholesterol 3mg		**1%**
Sodium 130mg		**5%**
Total Carbohydrate 3g		**1%**
Dietary Fiber 0g		0%
Sugars 1g		
Protein 8g		
Vitamin A 40%	•	Vitamin C 2%
Calcium 0%	•	Iron 0%
*Percent Daily Values are based on a 2,000 calorie diet. Your daily values may be higher or lower depending on your calorie needs.		

✳ *Eat lean proteins.* By consuming only low-fat proteins, such as fish, beans, lean beef, poultry, game, and non-fat dairy, you will reduce the saturated fat in your diet, thereby reducing your risk for heart disease and cancer, because a diet high in saturated fat is linked to elevated cholesterol. Fish, because it contains the good omega-3 fats, does not need to be lean; the same is true for soy products that do not have added fat. Aim to limit red-meat protein sources to once a week or less.

Soy is truly a healthy food to eat and an excellent way to get protein without too much saturated fat. Research has shown that if you are in your early teenage years, during puberty, eating two to three soy servings per day can contribute a protective benefit against breast cancer. Soy has natural estrogen-like properties and contains isoflavones, natural plant compounds that protect cells against damage. There is ongoing research as to how the protective plant compounds in soy work in our system. According to recent research, the health benefits from the soy isoflavones found along with protein in natural soy products can help to decrease

✳
coach
tip

FINDING SOY WITH ISOFLAVONES

Soy Food	Isoflavones
Roasted soybeans, ½ cup	167
Green young soybeans, ½ cup	30
Soy protein isolate, dry, 1 ounce	57
Tofu, 4 ounces	38
Soy concentrate, dry, 1 ounce	12

While soy protein is healthy to eat, it may not always have isoflavones, because they can be lost during processing.

bone loss, reduce cholesterol (when 25 grams of soy protein were consumed), and aid in slowing the progression of prostate cancer.

If you would like to try soy, I recommend soy milk, young green soy beans from the pods, dry roasted soy nuts, soy burgers, or tofu as a start. Getting one to two servings of soy in a day contributes about 30 to 150 grams of protective isoflavones to your diet, which can be a healthy addition. However, if you are at risk for breast cancer, it is advisable to limit your soy intake to one serving a day until further research distinguishes whether the natural plant estrogens in soy can promote estrogen-based breast cancer.

At this point in time, while research is still young, I do not recommend that you take supplements of soy isoflavones. It is best to get your isoflavones with the naturally occurring protein it is attached to in the food.

* *Eat mainly whole grains, beans, and starchy vegetables.* Focus on whole foods (nonprocessed products) that have 2 or more grams of fiber per serving. Limit foods made with processed grains and flours. You can identify these products because they usually are made mainly of white starch or flour. Some of these foods include bread, pastas, cereals, white rice, powdered potatoes, and baked goods.

It is best to eat whole grains, beans, and legumes most of the time, because the fiber helps to slow down your digestion and thereby reduces the effect the grains or starches can have on your blood sugar. For example, a piece of whole-grain toast will take longer for your body to digest than a piece of white-bread toast. So, instead of your morning muffin, white-flour bagel, or cheese danish, reach for whole-grain toast, oatmeal, or other whole-grain cereal. Eating the high-fiber way will increase your energy, decrease your cravings, decrease your triglyceride levels, keep you "regular," and decrease your risk for diabetes and heart disease.

* *Eat five or more fruits and vegetables daily. Vegetables are unlimited.* You can get most of your essential vitamins and minerals from fresh fruits and vegetables, which are more readily absorbed by the body. One research study after another reports that people whose diets are rich in fruits and vegetables have lower incidences of heart disease, stroke, and cancer. Additionally, the dark green, orange, yellow, and red fruits and vegetables

coach

tip

Fiber requirements:

If you are under fifty years		If you are fifty years or older	
Men	38 grams of fiber/day	Men	30 grams/day
Women	25 grams/day	Women	21 grams/day

Based on the 2003 report of Dietary Reference Intakes by the National Academy of Sciences

Power Picks for Fruits and Vegetables

Cornell University reports that the produce with the highest protective benefits are:
Fruits—blueberries, red grapes, cranberries, apples, green grapes, oranges, grapefruit, bananas
Vegetables—garlic, broccoli, tomatoes, spinach, carrots, onions, green peppers

are high in antioxidant vitamins, which can prevent cell damage from oxidants.

Oxidants are highly reactive molecules produced by environmental influences, including stress, radiation, air pollution, smoking, and excessive oxygen in the body (caused by overexercising or by certain vitamins and minerals, such as iron). Oxidants can damage the cells of the body, which may result in wrinkled skin, cataracts, premature aging, arterial plaque, and, according to some researchers, certain cancers.

Recent research from Cornell University points to the protective benefits of additional plant compounds, called polyphenols, found in an individual vegetable or fruit. The findings at Cornell reveal that the nutrients in the fruits and vegetables work together to provide more benefit than any of the protective compounds can alone. So you are much better off eating the fruits and vegetables than assuming you will get everything you need in a supplement. See the sidebar for the most protective fruits and vegetables.

* *Supplement your diet with the following vitamins and minerals, unless you are consuming five or more servings of fruits and vegetables a day.* Food is the best source for any nutrient. However, supplements can be beneficial when you are having trouble eating a variety of foods daily. Supplements are recommended when you cannot eat five servings or more of different fruits and vegetables each day, and at least three servings of calcium-rich foods each day.

All supplements should be taken on a full stomach or with meals. An important fact to understand when taking supplements is that more is not necessarily better. Actually, too much of any one vitamin or mineral can inhibit the absorption of other essential nutrients. In addition, large doses of some vitamins and minerals are actually harmful. The guidelines provided by Active Wellness are safe levels of supplementation. Some brands of vitamins I recommend include Centrum, Solgar, and Twin Labs.

* *Multivitamin* (one multivitamin per day). It is best to take a multivitamin that contains 100 percent of the daily value for most vitamins and minerals. See below for specific guidelines for calcium, vitamin D, vitamin B$_{12}$, and iron.

In addition, if your multi does not contain the following antioxidants in the amounts listed, it can be helpful to take additional supplements to ensure that you are getting the benefits of the antioxidants daily.

* *Vitamin C* (250 mg per day).
* *Vitamin E* (100 IU per day). If you have high blood pressure, check with your doctor before taking a vitamin E supplement.
* *Selenium* (50 mcg per day).

Also, for disease prevention add the following B vitamin unless it is in your multi in the following amount:

* *Folic acid* (400 mcg per day).

* *Calcium and what goes along with it.* For every serving of calcium-rich dairy, juice, or soy foods you do not drink or eat, make sure your supplement contains 300 mg of calcium. (Refer to the chart of Calcium-Rich Foods on page 117.) If necessary, take an added calcium supplement that contains vitamin D, for optimal absorption.

If you are younger than fifty years of age and you follow the Active Wellness guidelines, you will be meeting your daily requirement of 200 IU of vitamin D. If you are over fifty years of age, a 400 IU of vitamin D is recommended daily, especially if it is not included in your daily supplement and you do not spend much time outdoors. If you are over sixty years of age, make sure your supplement contains 25 mcg of vita-

The coach tip box reads:

coach tip

Please see a Registered Dietitian or E-mail me at *www.activewellness.com* before deciding to take other supplements that provide more than 100 percent of the recommended dietary allowances (RDA).

min B$_{12}$—if not, consider taking a supplement. If you are seventy years of age or older, take 600 IU of vitamin D daily.

Caution: If you currently have or are at risk for heart disease, or if you are a male, make sure that your multivitamin does *not* contain iron. Recent research indicates that iron, an oxidizing agent, may increase your risk for heart attack. If you are a female and a vegetarian or peri-menopausal, supplemental iron is usually not a problem.

✳ *Eat low-fat and fat-free sweets sparingly and greatly reduce or eliminate high-fat desserts from your diet.* Most sweets and desserts provide only "empty" calories—that is, they do not contain many nutrients but do contain plenty of sugar and butter (saturated fats). Believe it or not, eating sugary foods can make you feel tired, low in energy, and hungry. The sugar in the foods is quickly digested by your body, elevating your blood-sugar levels, giving you an energy boost, often called a "sugar high." But that energy is short-lived. Since sugar is fuel for your body, your body works to absorb it by releasing the hormone insulin, which helps your body deposit the sugar to be used as energy in your cells. An hour or so later, your blood-sugar levels inevitably decrease, because the sugar in your blood has all been absorbed, and your energy will drop. Now, here's the kicker: Insulin works so well in taking in sugar, you are usually left with less sugar in your blood than you started with. This makes you feel tired and low in energy. At this low end of the sugar cycle, people often feel hungry and crave another sugary snack to give them another energy boost, or they reach for caffeine for a pick-me-up, thus starting the (vicious!) cycle again. Over the course of the day, your energy cycles downward with each peak and drop from sugar, leaving you exhausted by 6 P.M. You can avoid the sugar cycling by making a policy of eating a sweet only after a meal. When you eat this way, the meal acts as a buffer and slows down the rate at which the sugar is absorbed into your system.

✳ *Eat polyunsaturated and monounsaturated fats. Avoid saturated fats. Eliminate hydrogenated fats and fried foods.* Not all fats are bad for you. In fact, some fats are essential to good health. These "good" fats help to build and maintain cellular tissue, transport vitamins, and manufacture hormones. The chart below will help you distinguish between "bad" and "good" fats.

Saturated fat is the most prevalent fat in the American diet and is a leading contributor to high cholesterol levels, fatty plaque deposits in the coronary arteries, and cardiovascular disease in general. Saturated fats come from animal sources and are solid at room temperature. They include butter, lard, full-fat cheese, and the marbling in meat.

Hydrogenated fats are liquid oils made solid by the addition of hydrogen, as in margarine. They typically appear in shortenings, baked goods, cereals, snack foods, and fast foods. Once presumed "healthier" than saturated fats, current research indicates that hydrogenated fats raise total blood cholesterol levels and LDL cholesterol. In terms of your health, hydrogenated fats (margarines) are just as bad if not worse than saturated fats (butter).

Additionally, when fats are hydrogenated they produce a very damaging form of fat called trans-fatty acids. Trans-fatty acids create damaging free radicals that cause damage to our cells and arteries. Free-radical damage also caused by oxidants has been linked to cancer, heart disease, and premature aging.

Polyunsaturated and monounsaturated fats are the good "fats" and have a positive effect on your health. Both types come from plant sources, are liquid at room temperature, and have beneficial effects on blood cholesterol levels.

Polyunsaturated fats are noted for lowering total cholesterol levels and "bad" LDL cholesterol levels. LDL (low-density lipoproteins) is the "least desirable" to have at high levels, because it is the carrier that is responsible for depositing cholesterol on our arterial walls, creating plaque that can lead to a heart attack or stroke.

Monounsaturated fats not only lower total and LDL cholesterol levels but also appear to raise the "good" HDL cholesterol levels that are associated with a decreased risk of heart disease. HDL (high-density lipoproteins) are highly desirable because they are responsible for picking up cholesterol to be reused by the body. I like to think of them as "recyclers" that pick up waste (excess cholesterol) and carry it back to the liver to be reused. The more HDL you have, the better, because it will help clear the excess cholesterol from your system and reduce the problems that can be caused by your LDL cholesterol.

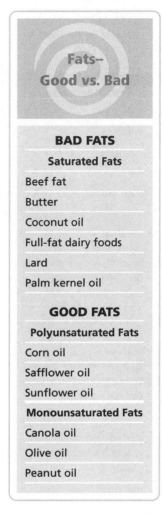

Fats— Good vs. Bad

BAD FATS

Saturated Fats

Beef fat

Butter

Coconut oil

Full-fat dairy foods

Lard

Palm kernel oil

GOOD FATS

Polyunsaturated Fats

Corn oil

Safflower oil

Sunflower oil

Monounsaturated Fats

Canola oil

Olive oil

Peanut oil

Essential fatty acids, also called omega-6 and omega-3 fatty acids, are part of the polyunsaturated fat family and are members of the "good" fats group. They are called essential, because the body cannot make them and must obtain them from foods.

Omega-3 fatty acids in particular have multiple beneficial effects on the body and should be eaten on a daily basis, since most American diets are deficient in them. Flaxseed is an excellent source of omega-3 fatty acids; one tablespoon contains 2,000 milligrams of omega-3. Among the many health benefits of omega-3 fatty acids, the major ones include lowering triglycerides, decreasing inflammation (and pain) in connective tissue diseases such as arthritis, and raising HDL cholesterol.

Omega-3 fatty acids can be found in many "fatty" fish. Try to add three servings of these fish foods to your diet each week. You can also get your omega-3 fatty acids from plant sources, including flaxseed, green leafy vegetables, canola oil, and especially soy products (soybeans, tofu, tempeh). The charts on the next pages list the fish, plants, and nuts that are the richest sources of omega-3 fatty acids.

Omega-6 fatty acids, which in the American diet are derived primarily from vegetable oils, are also essential to good health. Currently, they make up the greater percentage of essential fats in the American diet. Over the course of time, and with the development of technology for manufacturing oils, the American diet has become disproportionately high in omega-6 fatty acids, creating an imbalance.

Americans are not consuming enough omega-3 fatty acids. Currently, the ratio of omega-6 to omega-3 in the diet is about 10:1, but a healthful diet has a ratio of around 2:1—only two times the amount of omega-6 instead of ten times the amount. In order to create a healthful balance, it is important to make sure you are eating a greater amount of foods that are rich in omega-3 fats. You can do this by following the Active Wellness recommendation to increase omega-3-rich fish in your diet and to incorporate one tablespoon of flax meal per day or one teaspoon of flax oil into your diet. If you are a vegetarian, the flaxseed will help you meet recommended levels of omega-3 fats. The best supplement is the seed or flax meal, which can be sprinkled on salads, cereals, or yogurt. Capsules often go rancid, and for this reason they are not recommended.

Fish Rich in Omega-3 Fatty Acids

Based on a 3½-ounce serving: Contains 500 to 1,000 or more milligrams of omega-3 fatty acids.

Anchovies	Shark
Carp	Squid (calamari)
Coho (king, pink, sockeye)	Striped sea bass
Halibut	Swordfish
Herring	Trout, rainbow
Mackerel, Pacific	Tuna (albacore, bluefin)
Salmon (Atlantic, Chinook)	Turbot
Sardines, Pacific	Whitefish

Plant Sources Rich in Omega-3 Fatty Acids (not including nuts)

Based on the servings below, these plant sources contain 500 to 100 milligrams of omega-3 fatty acids.

Berries—strawberry, raspberry, blueberry (1 cup)	Soybeans, roasted (1 oz.)
	Soybeans, young green (½ cup)
Dark green leafy vegetables (e.g., spinach) (1 cup)	Tempeh (½ cup)
	Tofu (½ cup)
Dried beans (1 cup)	

✳ *Drinking six to eight 8-ounce glasses of water or water equivalents daily.* Over 60 percent of your body is water. For your body to function efficiently, it must be well hydrated. If you are trying to lose weight, drinking water also helps curb your appetite. Also, being dehydrated can cause headaches. If you are particularly susceptible to food cravings, especially cravings for sweets, a better alternative to eating is drinking water or flavored herbal tea from a "sipper" bottle. Sipping from a bottle is very satisfying and self-nurturing, echoing the comfort and nourishment we received through feeding as infants. I recommend you try it, particularly if you are trying to lose weight.

✳ *Reduce or eliminate caffeine from your diet.* This includes the caffeine in coffee, black tea, and colas. Decaf coffee and tea also contain small amounts of caffeine.

Your first cup of coffee can stimulate you to start your day, but did you know it can also make you more tired by day's end? Caffeine is a member of a group of drugs called methylxanthines, which can stimulate your appetite, act as a diuretic, and indirectly contribute to elevated blood cholesterol and blood pressure by inducing a stress response. The Caffeine Scale diagram below helps to show how caffeine works on your system.

Within five minutes after you drink your morning coffee, the caffeine begins to stimulate your central nervous system, triggering the release of stress hormones in your body, causing a stress ("fight or flight") response. The stress hormones are useful if you need to prepare yourself to fight or flee a dangerous situation, because the response readies your system by

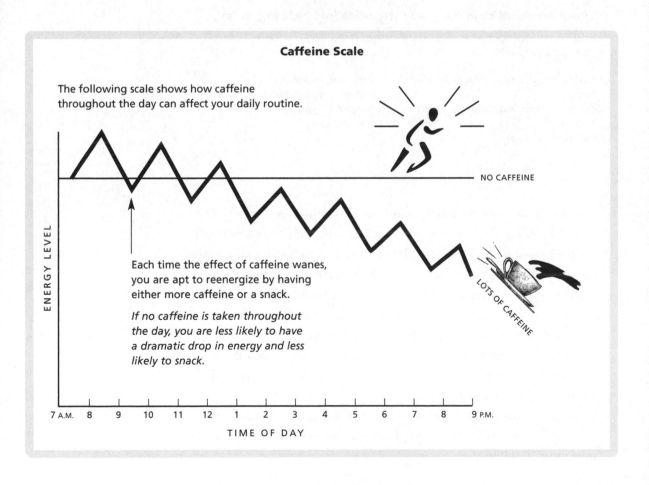

Caffeine Scale

The following scale shows how caffeine throughout the day can affect your daily routine.

NO CAFFEINE

LOTS OF CAFFEINE

ENERGY LEVEL

Each time the effect of caffeine wanes, you are apt to reenergize by having either more caffeine or a snack.

If no caffeine is taken throughout the day, you are less likely to have a dramatic drop in energy and less likely to snack.

7 A.M. 8   9   10   11   12   1   2   3   4   5   6   7   8   9 P.M.

TIME OF DAY

releasing sugars and fats into your bloodstream so your muscles have energy to run or fight. But if you are simply sitting at your desk you may feel a short charge of alertness, quickly followed by feelings of agitation. Within the next hour or so, after the stress response dissipates, you will probably feel more tired and hungry. At these low-energy times, many people reach for another cup of coffee or eat a snack that is often high in sugar to "pep up" and stay alert.

However, both caffeine and sugar only give you temporary feelings of increased energy, which quickly dissipate. For some people, this cycle of low energy followed by an infusion of caffeine or food continues the entire day, leaving them feeling exhausted and unable to focus by 3 P.M., because they are drained from the ups and downs in energy their body endured throughout the day. By eliminating caffeine, you will feel like you have more energy, because your energy level stays at an even level.

Caffeine also affects the body in many other unhealthy ways, including changing blood-sugar and triglyceride levels, increasing blood pressure and heart rate, constricting blood vessels, inducing anxiety, disrupting sleep patterns, and inhibiting the body's absorption of iron, zinc, calcium, potassium, magnesium, and sodium. In addition, caffeine has been linked to fibrous breast tissue and cardiovascular disease.

I strongly recommend that you eliminate the caffeine in your diet, particularly if you have heart disease, high blood pressure, or osteoporosis, or if you want to increase your energy and lower your stress level. Participants of the Active Wellness Program have been amazed at how energetic and calm they feel when they stop consuming caffeine. You can either eliminate all the caffeine in your diet right away, or slowly reduce the caffeine you consume over the course of several weeks. After two weeks of caffeine reduction, you can decide whether you feel like you have more energy and/or fewer cravings for sweets and refined carbohydrates.

To reduce the caffeine in your diet, start by determining where your caffeine is coming from. The chart below lists the levels of caffeine in a variety of foods and beverages. You can see that different beverages have different amounts of caffeine. Even decaf coffee has some caffeine, but far less than regular coffee.

Caffeine Content of Common Foods and Beverages

Source	Caffeine Content in Milligrams (mg)*	
Coffee (5-oz. cup)	**Range**	**Average**
Drip	60–180	115
Espresso	50–120	85
Percolator	40–170	80
Instant	30–120	65
Decaffeinated, brewed	2–5	3
Decaffeinated, instant	1–5	2
Tea (5-oz. cup)		
Iced (12-oz. glass)	67–76	70
Brewed (imported brands—black)	25–110	65
Brewed (U.S. brands—black tea)	20–90	40
Instant (1 tsp. powder)	25–50	35
Soft Drinks (12 oz.)		
Colas and diet colas	30–60	40
Cocoa and Chocolate Beverages		
Chocolate milk (8 oz.)	2–7	5
Cocoa beverages (5 oz.)	2–20	4
Solid Chocolate and Syrup		
Dark chocolate, semisweet (1 oz.)	5–35	20
Milk chocolate (1 oz.)	1–15	5
Bakers chocolate (1 oz.)	26	26
Chocolate syrup (1 oz.)	4	4
Coffee-flavored low-fat yogurt	45	45

Source: U.S. Food and Drug Administration and M. L. Bunker & M. McWilliams, "Caffeine Content of Common Beverages," *Journal of the American Dietetic Association,* Vol. 74, pages 28–32, January 1979.

When you eliminate or greatly reduce the caffeine in your diet, you may experience mild withdrawal symptoms, such as headaches, because caffeine is a mild drug. Aspirin can help with the headaches, and you will invariably feel better within three to four days. If you have been drinking large amounts of coffee or black tea (five or more cups per day), decrease your caffeine gradually by switching to a mix of half-regular and half-decaf coffee or tea. Drinking tea for the protective benefits of the naturally occurring plant compounds is a good idea, but to avoid the caffeine, stick to decaf green or black teas.

✳ *Avoid alcohol or drink in moderation.* Alcohol, like sugar, provides calories with little nutritional value. Excessive drinking of alcoholic beverages can cause health problems. A little alcohol goes a long way. Recent research reaffirms that moderate intakes of alcohol from wine, beer, and spirits can help protect against heart disease by reducing the stickiness of the blood and by interfering with blood clots. However, drinking moderate amounts of alcohol also has several downsides. Studies associating cancer with alcohol consumption have found that alcohol consumption may increase the risk of several cancers, including breast cancer, lung cancer, and cancer of the mouth, larynx, esophagus, and liver. Alcohol also stimulates the appetite and can alter your perception of how hungry you really are. So if you are trying to lose weight, consider avoiding alcohol as a good strategy. Furthermore, alcohol contains many calories and very little nutrition.

If you are a nondrinker, you should not start drinking to benefit your health. If you do drink and are concerned about its effects, weigh your personal risks and benefits. You should definitely avoid alcohol if you have very high triglycerides, uncontrolled hypertension, liver disease, breast cancer or risk of breast cancer, abnormal heart rhythms, peptic ulcers, or sleep apnea.

All the Active Wellness eating plans recommend that you limit yourself to one drink a day, equivalent to 5 ounces of wine, 12 ounces of beer, or 1½ ounces of distilled spirits (80 proof).

Stave Off Hunger and Curb Cravings

The reason many people get hungry on a low-fat diet is that they eat too many processed grains and starches that are typically made with white flour or contain a lot of sugar. These products don't make you feel full, and they can spike your blood sugar, perpetuating your hunger, so it is easy to overeat them. When you use the Active Wellness eating plans, you will be eating to maintain a more constant blood-sugar level, thereby giving yourself more energy and less dramatic bouts of hunger. To achieve this goal, incorporate the strategies below when you choose your foods each day.

Strategy 1: Mix Food Groups to Stay Full Longer

When you mix protein, carbohydrates, and fats together as a meal or snack your body will take longer to digest and absorb the nutrients from the food.

Carbohydrates are easiest to digest, followed by protein, and then fats. The sweeter the carbohydrate, typically the faster it is absorbed by your body. In the diagram on page 79, I have mapped out a general list of the types of carbohydrates. The carbohydrates at the top of the list are more likely to be absorbed quickly by your body and raise your blood sugar faster, which means if you eat them by themselves, they can trigger a "sugar high," which may increase your appetite. The less sweet and the less processed the food and the more fiber it has, the slower its rate of digestion, and the less likely it is to stimulate your appetite after you eat.

You can eat the foods at the bottom third of the carbodydrate list by themselves, since the fiber will help act as a buffer. But, if you think you are sugar sensitive or if you crave carbohydrates, it is best to mix carbohydrates from the top of the list (from sugar down to fruit) with either good fats and/or protein whenever you eat. And it is best to have your sweet after a meal so that the meal acts as a buffer and slows down the rate at which the sugar is absorbed by your body. Using this strategy will prevent the peaks and valleys of energy and hunger that can increase appetite and create cravings.

Like protein and fat, fiber also can help slow down the rate at which carbohydrates are absorbed into your system. It is for this reason that vegetables, while they are carbohydrates, are last on the list in relation to how they

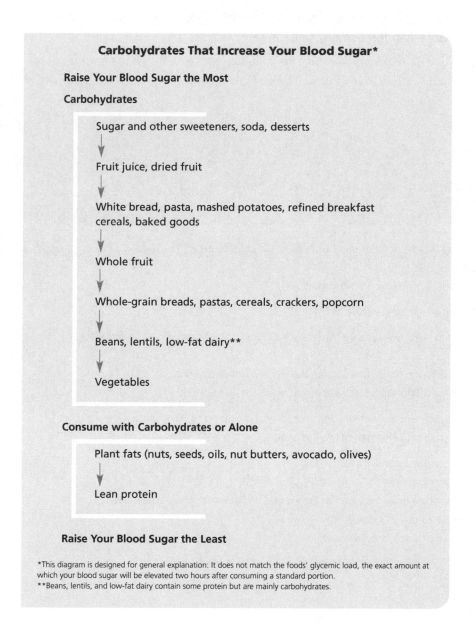

Carbohydrates That Increase Your Blood Sugar*

Raise Your Blood Sugar the Most

Carbohydrates

Sugar and other sweeteners, soda, desserts

Fruit juice, dried fruit

White bread, pasta, mashed potatoes, refined breakfast cereals, baked goods

Whole fruit

Whole-grain breads, pastas, cereals, crackers, popcorn

Beans, lentils, low-fat dairy**

Vegetables

Consume with Carbohydrates or Alone

Plant fats (nuts, seeds, oils, nut butters, avocado, olives)

Lean protein

Raise Your Blood Sugar the Least

*This diagram is designed for general explanation: It does not match the foods' glycemic load, the exact amount at which your blood sugar will be elevated two hours after consuming a standard portion.
**Beans, lentils, and low-fat dairy contain some protein but are mainly carbohydrates.

raise your blood sugar. Vegetables are so low in carbohydrate and high in fiber that they are great to eat anytime. This is why they are unlimited on your eating plan. Since fiber is also found in whole grains and on the skins and seeds of fruits, when you eat these types of foods, your blood sugar raises less than if you eat processed grains and fruits or juice.

Strategy 2: Limit the Amount of Processed Grains and Fruits You Eat to No More than Three at Any One Time

To control the rate at which your blood sugar rises, watch the portions of car-bohydrates you have at one time. Doing this will help to control the rise of

---

Applying the Active Wellness Eating Strategies

7 A.M. Breakfast	Whole-grain toast with peanut butter or whole-grain cereal with nuts A piece of fruit A glass of skim milk or fat-free yogurt
10 A.M. Snack	1 serving of nuts with a piece of fruit
1 P.M. Lunch	Bean soup (lentil, white bean, black bean) and a salad with some fish or lean poultry or A sandwich with whole-grain bread, lean protein, lettuce, tomato Fruit or low-calorie, low-fat sweet (if you don't use it at dinner)
3–4 P.M. Snack	Fruit, vegetable soup, low-fat yogurt, or low-fat cheese on whole-grain crackers, and/or a small salad with oil-based or low-fat dressing
6–7 P.M. Dinner	Lean protein (fish, chicken, tofu, eggs) 2 or more vegetables 1 cup of whole-grain side, such as brown rice, couscous, or whole-wheat pasta Alcohol (your optional one drink) Fruit or low-calorie, low-fat sweet

Refer to your Daily Allowance Card to determine the amount of servings you can have in each food group.

your blood sugar from the carbohydrates you have eaten, so you stay satiated longer.

Strategy 3: Try to Eat Every Three Hours to Keep Your Blood-Sugar Levels Constant

Use your Daily Allowance Card to keep track of how much food you eat each day. The menu on page 80 applies the Active Wellness eating strategies to a day of eating. Notice that the snacks and meals are always a combination of foods. Note that vegetables make great snack options.

Well done! You have taken a monumental leap toward optimal Active Wellness with all the work you have done in Steps 1, 2, and 3. Now all you need to start eating right is tips on how to put your eating guidelines into practice when stocking your pantry, dining out, or traveling. It's time to see how easy it can be to live with your eating plan every day!

Main Points to Getting Started with Your Personal Eating Plan: Rethinking Food, Fat, and Calories

✔ Be clear about what are myths and what are truths about healthy eating and effective, sound ways to lose weight.

✔ Once you determine your weight goals, you can follow a few easy steps to uncover how much energy your body needs each day to achieve your ideal weight and a healthy body mass index.

✔ Using the Active Wellness system and Daily Allowance Card, you can determine how to effectively translate the energy your body needs into a balanced selection of foods to eat every day.

✔ The Daily Allowance Card helps you track your "bank account of food" daily so that you can determine how much food you spent each day on your plan and how much you have left. The system promotes flexibility with meal selection, so you can use it wherever you are.

✔ The Active Wellness Basic Food and Nutrition Guidelines provide you with the knowledge you need to truly eat a healthy diet that is based on fact uncovered by medical research.

✔ Staying satiated is a matter of learning a strategy of eating that is based on how your body digests carbohydrates, proteins, and fats. When you eat this way, you don't get hungry between meals.

FACTORS IN FOODS THAT AFFECT BLOOD SUGAR

Other factors in the food composition can affect the rate at which the particular food will affect your blood-sugar levels.

Ripeness: The more ripe a fruit, the sweeter, and the higher sugar content it has.

Structure (Processing): Finely ground flour or applesauce affects your sugar more than coarsely ground flour or the whole apple.

Testimonial

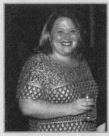

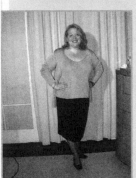

I started Active Wellness because I was looking for something that was more than just a diet. Active Wellness appealed to me because it involved not just eating, but exercise and stress management as well. Instinctually, I knew I needed to address all aspects of my lifestyle. My job was very stressful, I was working eight-hour days, my energy was low, and I was gaining weight. I was at the point where I knew I needed to do something or I would be endangering my health.

Active Wellness gave me the opportunity to address all aspects of my lifestyle. I started first with the eating program. Other programs I tried hadn't worked for me long term, so I was ready for a new program. Gayle's system, using the Daily Allowance Cards, really helped me get a true sense of what I was eating. I was surprised how easy it was to learn. Every time I would check off a serving, I would get a sense of satisfaction that I was doing something good for myself by eating right. While other friends were going on the fad diets of the time and looking unhealthy because of it, I felt good sticking to Active Wellness, because it made sense for my health, not just for my weight.

I now know how much food my body needs and in what proportions, so I can go to parties and dine out with friends at a restaurant and I can still follow my program without worrying about gaining weight. As I have lost weight and lowered my cholesterol, I have taken great pride in the fact that it has been my own food choices that have helped me to succeed. Looking back, I can see how much my bad habits of not making time for myself and skipping lunch had drained me of valuable energy I needed to perform my best at work and feel good about my weight. In the past, when I would skip lunch, I would eat twice as much as I needed at dinner. Not having time for exercise, this extra food quickly added up to extra pounds.

I still have to watch that the time I spend at the office doesn't take away from my Active Wellness Program, but I feel much more in control now. I don't know how I can live any other way and feel good about myself, and I have the balance in my life I was seeking.

(continued)

Now that I have my eating plan under control, my focus is on making sure I integrate exercise on a regular basis. In just six weeks on my exercise routine, I have dropped three dress sizes. The next step is integrating a more consistent exercise routine. I feel great! I know now that I can achieve my goal weight, because I have a plan that I have adapted to fit my own routine, it's flexible, and I know I can continue with it.

Susan, age thirty-seven, lost 30 pounds, dropped 3 dress sizes, decreased cholesterol 20 points . . . and still going

coach tip

QUICK AND EASY WAYS TO ESTIMATE SERVING SIZES

Use your hands to help you:

- One handful equals about half a cup; two hands together equals about one cup.
- One ounce of protein is typically equal to the width and length of your pointer and middle finger together or one slice of deli meat the size of your hand.
- The amount of animal protein you need each day is usually equal to the size of the palm of your hand, which does not include your fingers.
- One ounce of cheese is about equal to the length and width of your thumb if it is cubed or one piece if it is sliced.

Active Wellness Guide to Foods and Serving Sizes*

The Grains/Starches Group

(Bread and bread alternatives; cereals; starchy vegetables; pasta; rice and other grains; beans; crackers and snacks)

Note: Each grain/starch serving contains approximately 80 calories, 15 grams carbohydrate, 3 grams protein, 0 to 1 gram fat, 2 grams fiber.

Food	Equivalent of One Active Wellness Serving
Bread and Bread Alternatives	
Bagel, large	¼ bagel = 1 ounce
Bagel, small (mini)	½ bagel = 1 ounce
Bagel stick	½ bagel stick = 1 ounce
Bread, reduced calorie	2 slices = 1 ounce
Bread (whole-wheat, whole-grain)	1 slice = 1 ounce
Breadcrumbs	1 ounce = 4 tablespoons
Breadstick, crisp	1 ounce = 4 tablespoons
Dinner roll	1 small roll
Egg-roll wrapper (not fried)	1 wrapper
English muffin	½ muffin
Hamburger bun (whole-wheat, whole-grain)	½ bun
Hard roll (whole-wheat, whole-grain)	½ roll

Low-fat muffin (blueberry, banana, etc.)
    3-ounce muffin (small)
    6-ounce muffin
	
	½ muffin
	¼ muffin

Pancakes (4 inches across)	2

Pita bread (whole-wheat, oat, whole-grain)
    Mini
    Medium
    Large
	
	5 pitas
	1 pita = 1 ounce
	½ pita

Tortilla (corn or whole-wheat)	

*Servings are adapted from the American Diabetes Association and the American Dietetic Association Exchange Lists for Meal Planning.

Bread and Bread Alternatives (continued)	Equivalent of One Active Wellness Serving
6-inch tortilla	1 tortilla
8-inch tortilla	1 tortilla
10- to 12-inch tortilla	½ tortilla
Waffles	1
Wonton wrapper	4
Cereals	
Cereal, dry (puffed)	1½ cups
Cereal, dry (whole-grain, without nuts)	1 cup or serving equivalent listed on box
Cereal, hot	1 pack of instant or 1 cup cooked
Unprocessed bran	⅓ cup
Wheat germ	3 tablespoons
Starchy Vegetables	
Corn	One 6-inch corn on the cob or ½ cup cooked
Peas	½ cup cooked
Plantains	½ cup cooked
Potatoes (white, sweet, yams)	½ medium potato or ½ cup cooked
Winter squash (butternut, acorn, etc.)	½ cup cooked
Pasta, Rice and Other Grains, and Beans (Cooked and Uncooked)	
All pasta, rice and other grains, and beans (cooked in water or broth)	½ cup cooked
Bean soup	1 cup
Miso (soy product)	3 tablespoons or 1 cup of miso soup
Crackers and Snacks	
Bavarian, hard pretzel	1 large
Graham crackers	6 sections
Other crackers	Refer to serving equivalent listed on package
Popcorn, lite (packaged)	1 ounce = 1 cup
Popcorn, plain (air-popped or low-fat)	3 cups

Crackers and Snacks (continued)	Equivalent of One Active Wellness Serving
Potato or tortilla chips (fat free)	1 ounce = 1 cup
Rice cakes	2 large or 6 mini
All other low-fat snacks	Use serving equivalent listed on package

Vegetables

Each vegetable serving contains approximately 25 calories, 5 grams carbohydrate, 2 grams protein, 0 grams fat, 2 grams fiber.

Note: You may eat an unlimited number of vegetable servings (except for the starchy vegetables listed under Grains/Starches). You may use fresh or frozen vegetables, as long as they are prepared without added fat. However, vegetable juice and tomato sauce should be limited to two servings per day. For purposes of keeping track of the number of units you eat, one serving of vegetables is equivalent to the following:

Food	Equivalent of One Active Wellness Serving
Cooked vegetables	½ cup
Raw vegetables	1 cup
Tomato sauce	½ cup = 4 ounces
Vegetable juice	1 cup = 8 ounces

Proteins

Note: Try to eat mostly protein foods from the lean category. If you are a vegetarian, this rule does not apply.

Lean Protein
Each ounce of lean protein contains approximately 55 calories, 0 grams carbohydrate, 7 grams protein, 1 to 3 grams fat, 0 grams fiber.

Food	Equivalent of One Active Wellness Serving
Beans, dried or split peas	½ cup cooked
Beans, pureed (e.g., hummus)	⅛ cup = 2 tablespoons
Bean soup	½ cup
Egg substitute	¼ cup

Lean Protein (continued)	Equivalent of One Active Wellness Serving
Egg whites	2
Fish	1 ounce cooked
Game duck, pheasant (no skin), goose, rabbit, venison, buffalo, ostrich	1 ounce cooked
Lean beef (flank, round, sirloin, top loin), tenderloin, roast (rib, chuck, rump), steak (porterhouse, cubed, T-bone), trimmed of all visible fat (USDA Select or Choice grades)	1 ounce cooked
Lean ham, Canadian bacon	1 ounce cooked
Pork, fresh ham, tenderloin, center loin, sirloin, trimmed of all visible fat	1 ounce cooked
Poultry, chicken, or turkey (skinless)	1 ounce cooked
Shellfish	1½ ounces cooked
Soy products (fat-free)	See nutrition facts label on package
Textured vegetable protein	1 ounce cooked
Veal, trimmed of all visible fat	1 ounce cooked
Vegetarian burgers, hot dogs (fat-free, low-fat)	1 serving cooked

Medium-Fat Protein

Each ounce of medium-fat protein contains approximately 75 calories, 0 grams carbohydrate, 7 grams protein, 5 grams fat, 0 grams fiber.

Note: Use these foods for vegetarian protein sources.

Food	Equivalent of One Active Wellness Serving
Baked tofu, tempeh	¼ cup = 2 ounces
Meat analogs (low-fat)	See nutrition facts label on package
Tofu, tempeh	½ cup = 4 ounces
Whole egg	1

Fruits

Each fruit serving contains approximately 60 calories, 15 grams carbohydrate, 0 grams protein, 0 grams fat, 2 to 3 grams fiber.

Food	Equivalent of One Active Wellness Serving
Fresh or Frozen Fruit	
Bananas	½ large or 1 small
Cherries	10 (1 handful)
Fresh berries	1 cup
Fresh fruit	1 piece (the size you can hold in one hand)
Grapefruit	½
Grapes	15 (1 handful)
Honeydew	2-inch slice = 1 cup cubed
Melon, cantaloupe	⅓ melon = 1 cup cubed
Pineapple	¾ cup cubed
Watermelon	1-inch slice, 1¼ cups cubed
Fruit Juices	½ cup = 4 ounces
Dried Fruits	
Apple halves	4 slices
Apricot halves	8 halves
Dates	3
Figs	1
Prunes	3 medium
Raisins, cherries, cranberries	2 tablespoons

Dairy

Each dairy serving contains approximately 100 calories, 12 grams carbohydrate, 8 grams protein, 0 to 3 grams fat, 0 grams fiber.

Note: May be exchanged for soy-based or rice-based dairy alternatives.

Food	Equivalent of One Active Wellness Serving
Milk	
Buttermilk, low-fat	1 cup = 8 ounces
Evaporated, skim	½ cup = 4 ounces
Milk, skim (nonfat, can be protein fortified) or low-fat (1%)	1 cup = 8 ounces
Nonfat dry milk powder	⅓ cup
Nonfat or low-fat yogurt	1 cup = 8 ounces
Rice milk, nonfat or low-fat	1 cup
Soybean milk, nonfat or low-fat	1 cup
Cheeses	
Cottage cheese	½ cup
Hard cheese, low-fat (less than 3 grams of fat per serving)	1½ ounces
Hard cheese, lite (4 grams of fat or less)	1 ounce
Parmesan cheese, grated or shredded	2 tablespoons
Ricotta, low fat or fat free	½ cup

Fats

Each fat serving contains approximately 45 calories, 0 grams carbohydrate, 0 grams protein, 5 grams fat, 0 grams fiber.

Note: A certain amount of fat is necessary in everyone's diet. The "trick" is to choose your fat servings carefully, so that you use it where you will most enjoy it. For your health it is ideal to eat most if not all of your fats from plant sources. Here are suggestions for doing just that. On the next page are servings for foods high in unsaturated fats ("good fats").

Food	Equivalent of One Active Wellness Serving
Oils	
Monounsaturated:	
Canola, olive, peanut	1 teaspoon

Oils (continued)	Equivalent of One Active Wellness Serving
Polyunsaturated:	
Corn, safflower, sesame, soybean, sunflower, walnut	1 teaspoon
Nuts and Seeds	
Almond butter	1 teaspoon
Almonds	6
Cashews	6
Chestnuts, Chinese (water)	6
Chestnuts, European	6
Hazelnuts	1 tablespoon
Macadamia nuts	1 tablespoon
Peanut butter, natural	2 teaspoons
Peanuts, small	20
Pecans	4 halves
Pine nuts	15
Pistachios	15
Pumpkin seeds	1 tablespoon
Sesame seeds	1 tablespoon
Sunflower seeds	1 tablespoon
Soy nuts	2 tablespoons
Tahini (sesame paste)	1 teaspoon
Walnuts	4 halves
Most other nuts	1 tablespoon
Most other nut butters	1 teaspoon
Other Fats: Dressings, Condiments, and Miscellaneous	
Avocado	2 teaspoons = ⅛ fruit (1 ounce)
Cream cheese, low-fat	1 tablespoon
Creamers, powder or liquid	1 tablespoon
Mayonnaise, fat-free, low-fat	1 tablespoon
Mayonnaise, soy, low-fat	1 tablespoon
Olives, black (large)	8
Olives, green (small)	10
Salad dressing, regular (no cream)	1 tablespoon

Other Fats (continued)	Equivalent of One Active Wellness Serving
Salad dressing, low-fat	2 tablespoons
Sour cream, low-fat	¼ cup = 4 tablespoons

Sweets/Desserts

Each sweets serving contains approximately 100 calories, 18 grams carbohydrate, 0 grams protein, 0 to 3 grams fat, 0 to 2 grams fiber.

Note: Enjoy your sweets, but be aware that they provide very little nutritional value. Sweets may also promote sweet cravings.

Food	Equivalent of One Active Wellness Serving
Cake or fruit pie (less than 3 grams of fat per serving)	One ½-inch-wide slice
Cookies (less than 3 grams of fat per serving)	2
Granola bars, fruit bars	½ bar
Low-fat ice cream	4 ounces = small serving
Nonfat frozen yogurt	4 ounces = small serving
Nonfat frozen yogurt with fat-free hot fudge	3 ounces yogurt plus 2 tablespoons fudge
Other low-fat or fat-free desserts	See serving size on package.

Alcohol

Each alcohol serving contains approximately 100 calories, 0 to 12 grams carbohydrate, 0 grams protein, 0 grams fat, 0 grams fiber.

Note: Alcohol can be enjoyable, but limit yourself to one serving a day. More can be harmful to your health.

Beverage	Equivalent of One Active Wellness Serving
Beer, light	12 ounces
Distilled spirits (80 proof)	1½ ounces
Wine	5 ounces

Water or Water Equivalents

Note: Everyone should try to replenish their body with six to eight 8-ounce glasses of water per day.

Beverage	Equivalent of One Active Wellness Serving
Bouillon, broth, consommé	8 ounces = 1 cup
Club soda	8 ounces = 1 cup
Herbal teas, hot or cold	8 ounces = 1 cup
Mineral water	8 ounces = 1 cup
Seltzers, flavored but unsweetened	8 ounces = 1 cup
Tonic water, sugar-free	8 ounces = 1 cup
Water	8 ounces = 1 cup

Foods to Use Sparingly

Note: The foods listed below do not have to be tallied on your Daily Allowance Card. Use them sparingly throughout the day, up to three times per day.

Food	Equivalent of One Active Wellness Serving
Sweeteners	
Honey	1 tablespoon
Maple syrup	1 tablespoon
Molasses	1 tablespoon
Sugars	1 teaspoon
Condiments and Spreads	
Cocoa	1 tablespoon
Cream cheese, fat-free	1½ tablespoons
Fruit jam, naturally sweetened	1 tablespoon
Horseradish	1 tablespoon
Ketchup	1 tablespoon
Mayonnaise, fat-free	1 tablespoon
Mustard	1 tablespoon
Oil spray	2 to 3 sprays
Sour cream, fat-free	2 tablespoons

Foods to Use Anytime

Note: Food items that have an asterisk can be high in sodium.

Bouillon or broth*

Flavoring extracts

Gelatin, unflavored or sugar-free

Herbs, seasonings, and spices

Marinades, fat-free*

Salad dressing, fat-free*

Sauces, fat-free (e.g., Tabasco, Worcestershire)*

Tea, herbal

Counting Combination Foods

There are many foods that are combinations of several food groups, such as pizza, lasagna, or stew. If the meal is made with low-fat ingredients, you can determine how to check it off on your Daily Allowance Card by considering all the servings of food groups that were combined to create the meal.

For example: 1 slice of cheese pizza (thin crust) is made with the following ingredients: the crust (approximately 1½ servings Grains/Starches group) + tomato sauce (Vegetable group) + mozzarella (2 servings Dairy group) + 2 fat (an extra fat for each serving of regular fat mozzarella).

For frozen meals you can either use the exchange list on the package or treat them as a combination food and decipher the different food groups that the meal contains.

Please Note: If you do not see a food item you desire on the list, determine the food category in which it belongs and compare its nutrition information with the requirements for calories, carbohydrate, protein, and fat listed in the Active Wellness food list. If the food item is comparable in energy nutrients and calories, feel free to use it in your eating plan.

Starter Eating Plan

General Eating Plan and Vegetarian Eating Plan for Women and Men

(Please note that additional servings are given for men.*)

Breakfast

1 Grains/Starch	1 cup dry-flake whole-grain cereal or hot cereal, or 1 slice whole-grain toast
1 Fruit	1 cup berries or 1 piece of fruit your choice
½ Dairy	½ cup skim milk or low-fat soy milk
Water Equivalent	1 to 2 cups herbal tea or water
*Men add: 1 Grains/Starch	1 cup dry-flake whole-grain cereal or hot cereal, or 1 slice whole-grain toast
Other	Vitamins
Other	Sprinkle flax meal on cereal (already counted as part of plan)

Snack

Water Equivalent	1 cup hot herbal tea
2 Fats	1 handful nuts (about 12 large nuts, or 40 peanuts)

Lunch

1 Grains/Starch	½ cup cooked beans (e.g., chickpeas, kidney beans, black beans, lentils) or 1 cup bean soup
1 Fat	2 tablespoons low-fat salad dressing
Vegetables (Free) Equals about 3 servings of vegetables	Large salad w/ dark green lettuce or spinach, ½ cup other vegetables that are unlimited—can include carrots, tomatoes, plus any other vegetables you would like
1 Sweet	½ cup low-fat or fat-free frozen yogurt
Water Equivalent	2 cups (16 ounces) herbal tea, water, or sparkling water
*Men add: 2 Grains/Starch	½ cup bean salad (if oil is added to the salad—count as a Fat) or ½ cup pasta salad or potato salad with fat-free or low-fat dressing, or 1 ounce popcorn or low-fat or fat-free chips; or use the two grains for whole-grain bread and make a sandwich with your protein. Use veggies on sandwich and as a side salad or soup.
1 Fat	1 tablespoon nuts or seeds
2 oz. Protein	2 ounces lean protein (e.g., fish, shellfish, chicken breast, turkey breast)

Snack

1 Fruit	1 small apple or orange or other fruit of choice
1 Dairy	1 cup (8 ounces) low-fat or fat-free yogurt
Water Equivalent	2 cups (16 ounces) herbal tea, water, or sparkling water

Starter Eating Plan (continued)

Dinner

4 servings lean protein equivalent	4 ounces lean poultry, fish, beef, pork, or 6 ounces shellfish, or 2 cups tofu— don't hesitate to use a sauce or marinade to add flavor.
*Men add: 1 serving to make a total of 5 servings	
1 Grains/Starch	1 cup any cooked grain: brown rice, whole-wheat couscous, barley, whole-wheat grain pasta
*Men add: 2 Grains/Starch	1 cup bean soup plus an extra serving cooked grain (½ cup) or 2 slices bread or 1 cup cooked grain or a whole baked potato or sweet potato
1 Vegetable	½ cup steamed broccoli
2 Vegetables	Mixed salad (2 cups raw vegetables) or 2 more cooked vegetables
2 Fats	2 tablespoons low-fat salad dressing and 1 teaspoon oil (canola or olive oil for cooking)
1 Alcohol: If you do not drink, you can trade alcohol for an extra serving of anything	1 alcoholic beverage equivalent (e.g., 5 ounces wine), or 1 serving of fruit or grain (e.g., ⅓ cantaloupe melon or add an extra ½ cup cooked grain to your meal or 1 cup bean soup)
Water Equivalent	2 cups (16 ounces) sparkling water or herbal hot or iced tea
*Men add: 1 Fruit	1 cup berries or other fruit

Snack

Water Equivalent	1 cup hot herbal tea
*Men add: 1 Grains/Starch	1 ounce whole-wheat pretzels or low-fat or fat-free popcorn

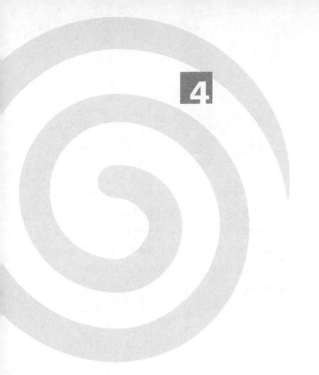

4

Putting Your Eating Plan into Practice Anywhere

Dining Out Made Easy

By using several simple strategies, dining anywhere while staying on your Active Wellness Program can be easy and satisfying. Know that different strategies are needed for different environments. In a restaurant, your goal is to take control of the food you order by asking questions and making creative choices from the menu. When you are with family, you may need to bring a dish you can eat and share with the group. Here are recommendations to follow depending on your particular situation.

The recommendations I've put together here come from the days when I was a chef and from my understanding of how a restaurant really functions, from the kitchen to the dining room. Here's an insider's tip: When you dine out, you are more in control than you think. You are the customer, and in the restaurant business, "the customer is always right." In fact, throughout the entire hospitality industry, the primary goal is to please the guest.

Dining Out in Restaurants

Ten Active Wellness Restaurant and Special Event Dining Strategies

① **First things first.** Don't go to the restaurant or party starving. If you know it is going to be a while before you eat dinner or have appetizers, have a late snack to curb your appetite—something light, such as a yogurt, salad, piece of fruit, or some nuts.

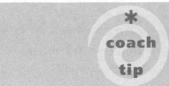

If a restaurant makes health claims on its menu items, that restaurant is required by law either to have nutrition information available as a reference for you to read or to use standard analyzed recipes from an organization such as the American Heart Association. Feel free to question how any dish is prepared and what ingredients it includes. Although the labeling law now exists, it is still new and up to you to be your own "food police."

2 **If you drink alcohol during the cocktail hour, start slowly or wait until your meal.** Alcohol can spur your appetite. Try beginning with a glass of sparkling water with a slice of lime or lemon added. No one will know this is not a drink. Or try mixing juices together with sparkling water (one quarter juice and three quarters soda water). This drink is both tasty and healthy and has more flavor than water with lemon or lime. You can also opt to have a weaker drink by mixing less alcohol with a low-calorie mixer. Saving your drink to have with dinner will limit the effect alcohol has on your hunger level.

3 **Be ready for the breadbasket.** When you sit down at a restaurant table, one of the first things the waiter or waitress does is put bread on your table. This can be a problem if you are one of those people who cannot control themselves around a breadbasket, especially when you're really hungry. Since bread is part of the grains/starches group, you can use your Active Wellness serving guidelines and count each slice of bread as one serving. But if you do that, remember that you then have less grain servings to eat at dinner.

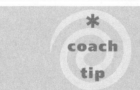

* coach tip

OTHER BREADBASKET STRATEGIES

If bread is one of the foods you tend to overeat, ask the server to take the bread-basket away. Call ahead and ask the restaurant to prepare a platter of crudités (fresh-cut vegetables) for the table, to be served as soon as you sit down. This gives you something to munch on while you are waiting for your dinner. Order a favorite beverage and slowly drink this instead of eating bread while you wait for dinner.

④ Mix and match from the entire menu, regardless of where the item is located. For example, if you want to start your meal with fresh fruit but it is listed under "Desserts," feel free to order it as an appetizer. Think of yourself as someone on a treasure hunt as you attempt to discover all the healthy options on a menu when making your meal selection. Then, find out whether you can make substitutions to the meal defined on the menu, so that it is more appropriate for your eating plan. For example, if a dish has a cream sauce, you can substitute a tomato sauce or wine sauce instead: Either of these sauces will be lower in fat.

If you can't find a healthy entrée on the menu, ask that the item be prepared using a healthier cooking method, such as steaming, baking, broiling, or grilling. Even light sautéing is better than frying. Have fun mixing and matching menu options. Who knows? You may discover a great new combination!

⑤ Make substitutions. Many Active Wellness participants have the best results in restaurants when they suggest the substitutions and modifications. On most occasions, when you let the chef know your health limitations, you'll be pleasantly surprised by what you are served. But at times when the kitchen is very busy, your best bet is to give the server

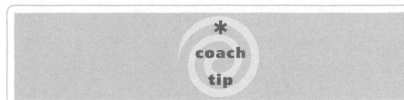

coach tip

FOR PARTIES

If you are at a dinner party, determine whether you want to make a meal out of the hors d'oeuvres or save yourself for the main meal. One good way to determine your eating strategy is to ask a server what the main entrée will be. Try to eat only one serving of several appetizers or make a meal of a favorite one: Don't load up on each type of appetizer. Do your best to estimate how the appetizers fulfill the option equivalents on your Daily Allowance Card.

specific instructions about how you would like the dish prepared in order to meet your requirements.

6 **Determine your hunger level and order appropriately.** Becoming absorbed in all the choices a restaurant offers is a common hazard. If your eyes are bigger than your stomach, you end up ordering more food than you need to satisfy your hunger. This tendency is dangerous for those who feel that they must eat everything on their plate. Ordering only the amount of food you want to eat at a given time is the wisest choice, so take your hunger level into account when you order your meal. If you are aware of how hungry you truly feel and you consider what food options remain on your Daily Allowance Card for that day, you'll gain a better sense of how much food to order.

Hunger Scale

The following scale is an easy way to determine your level of hunger at any given time. The *Decision Area* is where you should begin eating when you are hungry (4), and stop eating when you are satisfied (6).

1. **Starving**	So hungry you can eat the curtains (i.e., missing two meals or more).
2. **Extremely Hungry**	Consuming too few calories and missing meals.
3. **Very Hungry**	Missing a meal or waiting too long before meals (i.e., more than 5 hours).
*4. **Hungry**	Time to begin eating. Hunger should begin 4–5 hours from a meal. At this stage you have the most control and choice over what you eat.
5. **Not Hungry, Not Full**	Not yet satisfied but feelings of hunger are gone.
*6. **Satisfied**	You have eaten the appropriate portions of food.
7. **Full**	You can feel your stomach against your clothes.
8. **Very Full**	You feel the need to open your pants and pull at your waistband.
9. **Stuffed**	You are so uncomfortable that you feel as if you cannot move.
10. **Sick**	You feel physically ill; your stomach is in pain.

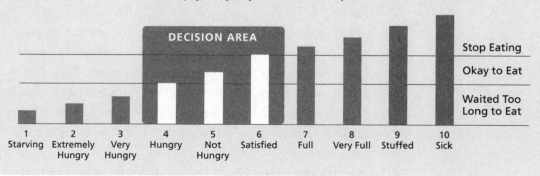

WHEN DINING OUT

Keep in mind that restaurants almost always serve double portions as entrées. So you typically can eat half of a meal, split one with a friend, or order an appetizer as a meal. When you do receive a large portion, plan to take some home for lunch the next day, or simply leave it. Remind yourself that leaving food on your plate is perfectly acceptable: You should eat until you are satisfied, not stuffed. Check in with the Hunger Scale to see where you are. Try not to eat too much, or wait too long to eat.

7 Use the "meal-layering" strategy. Meal layering helps you feel full on less food. The premise of meal layering is to use all the food groups to your advantage by ordering the lower-calorie and fiber-rich foods first, prior to your entrée. This is a strategy that is used at health spas, which can also be applied to dining out or eating in.

The way to meal-layer is to order a light appetizer or two, followed by your entrée. For example, have a light, broth-based soup and a salad with low-fat or fat-free dressing. This will help you to fill up on low-calorie, healthy food. It also begins the twenty-minute interval needed to signal your brain that food is now in your stomach, decreasing your feelings of hunger. If you eat most of your food before the twenty-minute mark, your body suddenly feels full after you may have already eaten too much. If you eat slowly and use the meal-layering strategy, you'll feel full on less food. Try meal layering at home. You'll be amazed at how well this method of eating works, and how easy it is to arrange. Meal layering is especially helpful if you're cutting portion sizes to lose weight and are accustomed to eating large quantities of food.

8 Always ask questions about how your food is prepared. The Dining Out Guides on page 105 suggest detailed questions, arranged by cuisine type. It is also important to let your server know you are concerned about your health before you ask questions about the food. The chef is the ultimate decision maker concerning what alterations in food preparation are possible. If your health needs are critical, your best strategy is to call the restaurant early and speak to the chef personally.

At restaurants, speak in terms of the ingredients, not the nutritional content. For example, when speaking about reducing the fat used to prepare a dish, refer to the type of fat that should be reduced: butter, oil, mayonnaise, or cream. Restaurants are notorious for adding butter to food in order to make it tender and moist. If you are concerned that added butter is a problem, ask them to limit all butter in the dish. If you are avoiding alcohol, any sauce that is prepared with alcohol still has alcohol in it after it is cooked—the alcohol does not completely burn off.

coach tip

KEY TERMS TO LOOK FOR ON THE MENU

Healthy preparations: baked, broiled, boiled, glazed, grilled, poached, steamed, seared, in broth

Healthy Ingredients: fresh, medallions (cuts of meat that are leaner), au jus ("with its own juice"), round and loin (cuts of meat that are leaner), marinated (usually adds flavor without fat, but ask about the ingredients, which may be high in sodium), beans, legumes, whole grains, vegetables, fruits, wine sauce

Ingredients typically high in sodium (avoid if you are following a low-sodium diet): chili sauce, smoked, cured, salted, cold cuts, hot dogs, sausages, pickled foods, salted crackers, snacks, salted nuts, anchovies, MSG, soy sauce, miso, meat tenderizers, capers, cheese, salt

If you have allergies to certain foods, don't forget to inquire whether a dish contains the specific ingredient that triggers your reaction. Don't be shy about asking questions; you're talking about your health. If you have many health concerns and need to ask questions and take your time going over the menu, plan to avoid the restaurant's rush hours when you dine out. Those hours tend to be 7 to 9 A.M. for breakfast, 12 to 2 P.M. for lunch, and 6 to 8 P.M. for dinner.

⑨ If you want dessert, think fruit. Dessert presents a tricky situation because many people have difficulty passing it up, particularly when with a group of people who all decide to order dessert. Desserts are usually loaded in calories because they are full of sugar and fat, which is why you would be wise to avoid them. A typical dessert at a restaurant can have 350 to 600 calories or more.

But never fear! The calories can be worked into your daily food options—a sweet serving is equal to 100 to 120 calories. Some healthy dessert selections are available; roasted or poached fruit, sorbets, angel food cake, hot soufflés, and low-fat ice cream or frozen yogurt all make good desserts. If you have to eat a regular dessert, the fruit desserts are often lower in calories than a rich chocolate dessert or cheesecake. Typically, a sliver or three spoonfuls of a higher-fat dessert will be equivalent to the calories in your sweet serving. Try to share your dessert with two or three people.

The dessert table, with its abundance of choices, provides great temptation to many people. The way to handle any large array of choices is planning what you'll take before you approach the table. Fruit should be your first choice. If you find yourself eyeing the pastries, ask yourself if they are really worth the calories. If not, perhaps you can wait for dessert until you go home. Then enjoy one of your favorite low-fat treats—without the guilt and extra calories!

⑩ Once you receive your food, enjoy it! This point is simple: If you have taken the effort to create a meal that you feel is right for your needs because you have asked the right questions, then when the meal arrives from the kitchen, enjoy it! Even if it contains one or two ingredients that are not quite right, still enjoy it. You did your best, and with each new restaurant experience, you learn more information that you can use the next time you dine out. Also, the more you return to the same restaurant, the easier time you'll have deciphering the menu and getting your food prepared the way you want it. Each restaurant's menu presents different challenges, but the process of studying the menu and asking questions is always the same.

Dining Out Guide 1

MEXICAN

Look for: Baked, Grilled, Sautéed, Soft Tortillas (Corn or Flour), Black Bean Soup, Salsa, Salads, Gazpacho Soup, Fajitas (without guacamole), Rice, Burrito (without cheese)

Watch out for: Fried, Excessive Cheese, Enchiladas, Refried Beans Flavored with Lard, Guacamole, Fried Tortilla Chips, Cheese Quesadilla, Sour Cream, Chorizo, Chiles Rellenos, Tacos, Flan, Sopapillas, Nachos, Chimichangas, Fried Ice Cream

Ask: Can you make this item with half the amount of cheese? Is this dish prepared with a lot of oil? If yes, can the oil be reduced?

CHINESE

Look for: Steamed, Baked, Stir-Fried (sautéed), Barbequed, Lots of Vegetables

Watch out for: Crispy, Fried, Batter-Fried, Pan-Fried, Breaded, Sweet and Sour, Egg Rolls, Spring Rolls, Peking Duck, Bird's Nest, Lo Mein, Scallion Pancakes, Combination Plate. If on a low sodium diet, watch out for the Soy Sauce and Hot & Sour Soup

Ask: Can you prepare this without MSG? Is this dish prepared with a lot of oil? If yes, can the oil used in preparation be reduced? Can this dish have extra vegetables added? May I have the meat, poultry, or fish steamed or stir-fried instead of batter-fried or deep-fried?

FRENCH

Look for: Poached, Steamed, Broiled, Roasted, Grilled, Provençal Cuisine, En Papillote, Sorbet, Vinaigrette, Au Jus, Marinated, Bouillabaisse, Demi Glacé

Watch out for: Crusted, Stuffed, Cheese (all types), "Light Sauce," Au Gratin, Béchamel, Béarnaise, Hollandaise, Beurre Blanc, Crème, Crème Fraîche, Crème Brûlée, Foie Gras, Pâté, Buttery, Gratiné, Pastry (all types), Gravy, Confit, Caesar Salad

Ask: Is this dish prepared with a lot of oil or cream? If yes, can the oil or cream used in preparation be reduced or omitted?

GREEK

Look for: Steamed, Baked, Roasted, Grilled, Mixed Vegetable Salads, Rice-Stuffed Grape Leaves, Pita Bread (without oil or butter), Roasted Eggplant, Soupa, Seafood, Tabbouleh, Plaki, Baba Ghanoush, Shish-Kabob, Olives.

Watch out for: Pan-Fried, Phyllo Dough, Tahini, Tzatziki (with full-fat yogurt), Goat Cheese, Hummus, Feta, Kasseri, Pastries (especially nuts), Lamb, Anchovies, Falafel, Locanico (sausage), Moussaka, Ice Cream

Ask: (If pita is served) May I have the pita without butter or oil? Is this dish prepared with a lot of oil/butter? If yes, can the oil/butter used in preparation be reduced or omitted?

INDIAN

Look for: Roasted, Marinated, Soup, Tandoori, Vegetables, Rice, Chapti, Naan, Tomatoes, and Onions

Watch out for: Fried, Pakora, Batter-Dipped, Somosa, Coconut/Coconut Milk, Ghee, Desserts, Cream Sauce, Lamb, Fritters, Rayta (with full-fat yogurt), Pappadams, Poori

Ask: Is the yogurt sauce made with full-fat yogurt? Is this dish prepared with a lot of oil/butter? If yes, can the oil/butter used in preparation be reduced or omitted?

ITALIAN

Look for: Baked, Broiled, Grilled, Roasted, Marinated, Sautéed, Polenta, Pasta, Half-Orders, Beans, Medallions, Vinaigrette, Tomatoes, Vegetables, Salads, Primavera, Fresh Clam Sauces, Mushroom Sauces, Vegetable Pizza Toppings, Seafood, Ham, Olives

Watch out for: Cream Sauces, Risotto, Alfredo, Four-Cheese, Extra Cheese, Fried Eggplant, Parmigiana, Pancetta, Carbonara, Francese, Milanese, Prosciutto, Tortellini, Piccata, Pepperoni, Salami, Meatballs

Ask: Is the eggplant fried? Is this dish prepared with a lot of oil/butter? If yes, can the oil/butter used in preparation be reduced? Are half orders of pasta available? Is this pizza made with part skim mozzarella or without cheese?

Never, never, never feel bashful about taking care of yourself by ordering healthy foods. What you eat 99 percent of the time makes the most difference in your overall health. An occasional deviation from your meal plan, on your birthday or another special occasion, is not terrible. But if you are following a low-fat diet because you have heart disease, even an occasional high-fat meal stresses your system and can cause problems. It would be wise to play it safe and stick to your healthy eating plan all the time.

Becoming an expert at deciphering menus the Active Wellness way doesn't take long. When you dine out, the anxiety of finding healthy foods on a menu is diminished. Food becomes a pleasurable part of the whole dining experience, rather than your sole focus. And when food becomes less of an issue for you, you'll feel more in control of your overall health.

Quick Meal Strategies for Eating on the Go

Some dining experiences are the "grab, eat, and run" kind. Often breakfast and lunch fall into these categories. During the day we typically run errands, have others to take care of, and do work, which leaves little time to prepare and eat meals. Eating becomes a matter of convenience. But remember that satisfaction remains important, regardless of how quickly or slowly you need to eat. And finding satisfying, quick meals is difficult unless you know where to look and what to do.

You have two main options for quick meals. One is to opt for prepared food that is available through home-delivery services, supermarkets, and home meal–preparation services. Your other option is to locate several food sources, including grocery stores, delicatessens, take-out emporiums, and pizza shops, that are close to your home or office. There is a chart on page 108 of some quick meals and how to count them on your eating program.

Setting Up Your Active Wellness Kitchen

One of the best ways to stay on your personal eating plan is to be prepared. Stocking your kitchen with the right foods makes healthy eating convenient and enjoyable.

Clean Out the Pantry

Action 1: Go through your cupboard, refrigerator, and freezer and remove all of the high-fat items, except actual fats such as oil and butter. Use as your guide the nutrition label on each product and discard any food that contains more than 3 grams of fat per serving. Any food product with 3 grams of fat or less per serving is considered a low-fat food; most of these are also low in saturated fats.

coach tip

Don't eat on the run! Sit down to eat every meal. Chew slowly and savor the scent, flavor, and texture of your food. Ask yourself questions to help you focus on the food: Do you like the flavor? Are you enjoying the eating experience?

coach tip

Don't forget, if a food is not low fat, you need to tally one extra fat per serving to account for the added fat and calories from the food.

Foods to Choose When You're on the Go

Foods	How to Count the Servings
Soups	
Bean soups (large bowl)	2 Grains/starches or 2 protein
Vegetable soup	Count as vegetables—unlimited
Sandwiches	
A lean meat sandwich (turkey, chicken breast, ham, lean beef) on 2 slices of bread	2 grains/starch, 4 servings of protein = 4 ounces, vegetables are unlimited
Wrap sandwiches	2 grains/starch, 3 servings protein, vegetables are unlimited
Cheese	1 slice of regular fat cheese = 1 dairy + 1 fat 1 slice of low-fat cheese = 1 dairy
Salads	
Greens and vegetables	Vegetables are unlimited
Meat, fish, poultry	1 large scoop at a salad bar = 2 protein
Tofu, beans	1 large scoop at a salad bar = 1 protein or starch
Hard-boiled egg	1 protein
Salad dressing	1 tablespoon oil and vinegar = 1 fat 2 tablespoons of low-fat dressing = 1 fat
Fruit Salad	Large chunks, 2 handfuls (1 cup) = 1 serving
Other Meals	
Roasted chicken (skin removed)	1 thigh or breast = 3 protein; 1 leg = 2 protein
Peel-and-eat shrimp, medium	3 to 4 shrimp = 1 protein
Yogurt, low-fat	8 ounces/1 dairy
Pizza with cheese, thin crust	1½ grains/starch, 2 dairy, 2 fat, 1 vegetable
Omelettes	3 protein, with cheese add 2 dairy and 2 fat, vegetables are unlimited
Burgers, lean beef, turkey	3 to 4 protein
Burgers, veggie	1 protein
Baked potato with vegetables and cottage cheese	2 grains/starch, 1 dairy, vegetables are unlimited
Burritos, with cheese, beans, rice, guacamole, no sour cream	4 grains/starch (2 for tortilla, 1 for rice, and 1 for beans), 2 dairy for cheese, 1 fat for guacamole

Fast-Food Healthy Picks

Below is a list of fast-food items and how to count them on your Daily Allowance Cards.

Restaurant	Calories	Servings per Item			
McDonald's					
Hamburger	280	2 Grains/Starches	1½ Protein	2 Fats	
Chicken McGrill w/o mayo	340	3 Grains/Starches	3 Protein	1 Fat	
Fruit 'n Yogurt Parfait w/o granola	280	1½ Grains/Starches	1 Dairy		1 Fruit
Kentucky Fried Chicken					
KFC BBQ Chicken Sandwich	260	2 Grains/Starches	4 Protein	1 Fat	
Corn on the Cob or BBQ Beans	150–190	2 Grains/Starches		½ Fat (only add for beans)	
Subway					
*7 Under 6™ Sandwiches	200–294	2 Grains/Starches	2½ Protein	1 Fat	1 Vegetable
*7 Under 6™ Salads	233–299	1 Grains/Starches	2½ Protein	1 Fat	2 Vegetables
*with meat or poultry					
Taco Bell					
Taco Bell Bean Burrito	380	3½ Grains/Starches	2 Protein	2½ Fat	
Arby's					
Light Menu Sandwiches	260–280	2 Grains/Starches	2½ Protein	1 Fat	
Salads with Chicken	160–210		3 Protein	½ Fat	3 Vegetables
Pizza Hut					
Veggie Lovers	220	1 Grains/Starches	1 Dairy	1½ Fat	1 Vegetable
Spaghetti w/Marinara	490	6 Grains/Starches			1 Vegetable

*Use reduced, low-fat or fat free condiments for all sandwiches and salads.

Action 2: Now go through your freezer and remove any prepackaged, frozen meals or side dishes that derive more than 30 percent of their total calories from fat. The nutrition label on prepackaged foods often lists the percentage of calories from fat. If it doesn't, you can easily calculate the percentage yourself by dividing the number of fat calories in a serving by the total number of calories per serving. Remember to check ingredients. If the fat is from plant or fish sources, it is good fat and okay to keep, even if it is above the "fat limit."

Action 3: Check all processed foods and discard any food that contains hydrogenated vegetable oil. Hydrogenated fats will be listed in the ingredients information on the package. Many prepared rice and pasta dinners come with flavoring packets that contain hydrogenated fats. These flavoring packets are often high in sodium as well. Discard the packets and keep the rice and pasta. The amount of trans-fats in a food product will soon appear on the nutrition facts label as required by the FDA, since the Institute of Medicine states that there is no safe level of trans-fats in the diet.

*
coach
tip

HOW TO CHECK YOUR FROZEN DINNERS TO MAKE SURE THEY ARE LOW IN FAT

Nutrition Facts

Serving size	1 meal
Calories per serving	500
Total calories from fat	125

1. Look at the calories per serving.
2. Find the calories from fat.
3. Divide the calories from fat by the number of calories per serving to determine if there is more than 30 percent calories from fat.

An example using the label information above:

This low-fat chicken dinner has 500 total calories per serving and 125 calories from fat. The percentage of fat from calories is 25 percent, as calculated by dividing the calories from fat by the total calories per serving: 125/500 = .25, or 25 percent. Since this chicken dinner meets the requirement, you can eat and enjoy it guilt free!

Action 4: Check your quantities of caffeinated beverages. Now is the time to rethink how many high-caffeine items you want to keep in the house, including espresso, dark-roast coffees, decaf coffee, black teas, and colas.

Restock the Pantry

When you begin the Active Wellness way of life, grocery shopping becomes fun, instead of a chore. You'll learn how to work your way around the market in record time because you'll be avoiding some food aisles completely.

Do plan to spend some extra time when you take your first Active Wellness shopping trip. You'll be reading the nutrition facts labels on all the items you purchase—checking for fat, sodium, and sugar contents. And you'll be looking for new food products that satisfy your plan's nutritional requirements.

One of the key facts to know about supermarkets, which will streamline your shopping time, is that all of the fresh-food items, including fruits, vegetables, fruit juices, meat, poultry, seafood, dairy, and sometimes even frozen food and bread products, are usually located around the perimeter of the store. Packaged and canned items are located in the center aisles of the store. Knowing this helps make healthy shopping easy and quick, since the majority of foods you will buy on a regular basis are fresh foods that are found on the outside aisles of the market.

✳
coach
tip

Farmers' markets are often good sources for fresh, ripe produce. If you have a weekly market in your area, try to take advantage of it. You may also find fresh produce stands and stores that are open year-round. It is usually worth the trip to these specialty produce markets, because you benefit by finding freshly picked produce that is often more flavorful.

Vegetables, fruits, and the starchy vegetables, which are members of the Grains/Starches group on your eating plan, are found primarily in the fresh produce section of markets. Vegetables and fruits are essential to good health and your daily eating plan. Pound for pound, they are the best supermarket buy. They add flavor, color, vitamins, minerals, and fiber to your meals and are invariably low in fat, sugar, and sodium. The most flavorful vegetables and fruits are those that are fresh and in season. Out-of-season produce usually is picked before it has ripened, and the ripening then takes place during shipping. Reducing the plant's natural aging process in this way also reduces both flavor and nutritional value. Keep in mind that the vegetable portions in your plan are minimum guidelines—fresh vegetables should be considered unlimited foods in your eating plan.

As you shop in the produce section, be adventurous and try some of the many unique varieties of fruits and vegetables that are now available. Fresh and loose produce is best, but if you are short on cooking time, you can buy prepackaged fruits and vegetables from the produce section or precut produce from the salad bar. This will save you preparation time at home. The special bags used for premixed salads and other fruits and vegetables help retain their freshness, but the food usually isn't as flavorful or as nutritious as loose produce. Both light and heat can enhance the loss of vitamins and

coach tip

An easy way to spot antioxidant-rich vegetables and fruits is to shop by color. Vegetables and fruits that are yellow, orange, red, and dark green generally pack the most nutrition per bite. See the antioxidant chart for specific fruit and vegetable suggestions.

coach tip

Fiber: When looking for fiber-rich fruits, a good rule of thumb is to buy those that have edible skins and seeds, such as apples and strawberries. Dried fruits are also high in fiber because they are dehydrated and therefore more concentrated. But eat them sparingly if you are watching your weight, because they are also high in calories.

Most vegetables are high in fiber. For best nutrition, avoid vegetables that are pale green, such as iceberg lettuce and peeled cucumber. Some fiber-rich vegetables and fruits include broccoli, carrots, Brussels sprouts, berries, potatoes with skin, apples, and corn.

Foods Rich in Antioxidants and Other Vitamins

Carotenoids	Vitamin C	Vitamin E	Folate
Vegetables			

Asparagus
Broccoli
Carrots
  Dark green,
  leafy vegetables
  (Arugula, Chicory,
  Dandelion Greens, Kale,
  Mustard Greens,
  Spinach)
Pumpkin
Tomatoes
	Broccoli
	Brussels Sprouts
	Cabbage
	Cauliflower
	Chili Peppers
	Dark green, leafy
	  vegetables (Collard
	  Greens, Kale, Mustard
	  and Turnip Greens)
	Peppers
	  (green and red)
	Radishes
		Artichoke
		Asparagus
		Broccoli
		Dark green, leafy
		  vegetables (Collard
		  Greens, Kale, Spinach,
		  Swiss Chard)
		Onions
			Asparagus
			Broccoli
			Beets
			Cauliflower
			Dark green,
			  leafy vegetables
			  (Collard Greens,
			  Kale, Spinach)
			Seaweed

Fruits			
Apricot Cantaloupe Mango Nectarine Papaya	Grapefruit Kiwi Orange Papaya Strawberries	Avocado Blueberries Mango Olives Papaya	Avocado Banana Blackberries Mango Papaya

minerals in foods. The produce section is also where you will find excellent vegetable protein sources, such as tofu and tempeh, low-fat salad dressings, along with fresh vegetable and fruit juices.

SALAD BARS

We tend to assume that salads are healthy, but the truth is that salads can be just as high in calories and fat as a typical fast-food meal. If you want to approach a salad bar with nutritional savvy, follow these healthy rules:

✳ If you like greens, choose the darkest salad greens that are offered, including romaine, leaf lettuce, and spinach. Or combine them for variety.

✳ Choose any other vegetables from the salad bar that you like, but if they are marinated in oil, don't forget to count fat servings, and if they are dressed with mayonnaise or fried, avoid them—they will typically be too high in fat to be worth eating.

✳ Make your salad by color: Don't forget that green, red, orange, and yellow vegetables are packed with protective nutrients.

✳ Fruit can be a sweet addition to your salad. It can add interest and flavor along with protective nutrients. So don't hesitate to add oranges, apples, or pears to your vegetables for variety.

✳ Look for protein sources to top off your salad, such as turkey breast, salmon, or chunks of chicken (without mayonnaise or oil); tofu; beans; and low-fat cottage cheese.

✳ Dress your salad with low-fat salad dressing; you get twice as much per serving as regular salad dressing. Or use olive oil and flavored vinegar, or balsamic vinegar.

✳ For dessert, have fresh fruit.

BUYING ORGANIC—IS IT BETTER?

Although it's difficult to determine whether organic produce is more nutritious, certified organic produce should contain less pesticide residue. The effects of long-term ingestion of pesticide residue are inconclusive, but it is always advisable to minimize your exposure when you can. Keep in mind, however, that organically grown products may not necessarily be pesticide-free, since airborne pesticides may drift onto organic produce from neighboring garden plots and farms. Also keep in mind that, even if organic produce isn't available, the benefits of eating fresh fruits and vegetables certainly outweigh any risk from pesticide residue.

FROZEN AND CANNED PRODUCE

Flash-freezing helps retain most of the nutritional quality of frozen produce, so frozen fruits and vegetables—without added sauces and sugars—are the best substitute for fresh produce. Frozen produce may be more nutritious than fresh, depending upon how the fresh produce has been handled and ripened.

Canned fruits and vegetables, packed in water, are available in low-sodium and low-sugar varieties. They are good alternatives to fresh produce. Look for canned fruits that are packed in water, not sugar syrup. Canned fruits retain most of their vitamin content, but canned vegetables may lose

coach tip

There are two types of fiber—insoluble and soluble. Think of the insoluble fiber as the outer skin that adds bulk to your diet and the inside of the plant as the soluble, which can help alleviate digestive problems and lower cholesterol. If you have trouble eating raw vegetables and fruits with skin, because of the fiber, cook your vegetables and peel the fruit.

You can identify organic produce by the USDA label, which verifies that the product is grown without conventional pesticides or petroleum-based fertilizers and the animal products are free of antibiotics and growth hormones.

The USDA Organic Seal will mean a product is either 95 or 100 percent organic—made from organic ingredients.

No Seal

Made with organic ingredients—products that contain 70 percent organic ingredients.

Some organic ingredients—products that contain less than 70 percent organic ingredients.

Other Claims

100% Natural: Food contains no chemical ingredients but is not organic.

NO GMOs: No genetically modified foods are used as ingredients.

Hormone free: Animals were not fed hormones.

some vitamins during the canning process, particularly vitamins B and C. Since these vitamins are often found in the liquid in which the foods are canned, use that liquid when you're cooking canned vegetables.

VEGETABLE AND FRUIT JUICES

Vegetable and fruit juices can help fulfill your eating plan's vegetable and fruit requirements. Vegetable juice makes a great snack. Check the labels on canned and bottled vegetable juices because some are high in sodium. V8 juice, as well as several other brands, now produce low-sodium vegetable juices. A wide variety of fruit juices are available, but check the nutrition labels carefully, as many contain as little as 10 percent real fruit juice. If the juice isn't labeled 100 percent fruit juice, it probably contains a high percentage of water and sugar, usually in the form of corn syrup. Avoid these fruit juices if you're trying to lose weight. Look for calcium-fortified orange juice to help meet your daily calcium requirement. Remember that fruit juice doesn't contain the fiber that fresh fruit does, so it won't fill you up as much as fresh fruit. One cup of vegetable juice and one-half cup of fruit juice are equivalent to one Vegetable and one Fruit serving, respectively.

DAIRY

At the dairy section, the simple rule of thumb to follow with all the products is that every dairy purchase you make should be low fat or fat free.

MILK Buy skim (nonfat) milk or 1 percent low-fat milk. A new type of milk on the market, "protein-enhanced skim milk," tastes as rich as whole milk but is actually skim. Local brands can be found in many supermarkets.

YOGURT Fat-free and low-fat yogurts are great snack foods, particularly if you are trying to boost your calcium intake. The best yogurts are those that have live bacteria cultures, which is marked on the container. Both organic and nonorganic yogurts, with or without fruit, are good choices. Many are also made with natural sweeteners, such as fruit juice, rather than refined sugars. If you are avoiding sweets, avoid the highly sweetened yogurts.

SOUR CREAM, CHEESES, AND SPREADS Sour cream now comes in low-fat and fat-free forms. Cabots' and Breakstone make excellent low-fat and fat-free sour creams. Good low-fat and fat-free cheeses are hard to find, no doubt about it, but finding them is not impossible. Several excellent-tasting brands of low-fat goat cheese and farmer cheese are on the market. Coach Farm makes a variety of delicious low-fat goat cheeses. Alpine Lace has a line of tasty low-fat and fat-free cheeses, along with several soft cheese spreads. Also, several low-fat and fat-free versions of American cheese are on the market. Although highly processed, they make good substitutes for their high-fat counterparts. Polly-O makes delicious fat-free and part-skim ricotta and mozzarella cheeses. Kraft makes both low-fat and fat-free Parmesan and cream cheese.

Calcium-Rich Foods

Food	Serving	Calcium (mg)
Yogurt, nonfat, plain	1 cup	452
Yogurt, low-fat, plain	1 cup	415
Yogurt, low-fat, vanilla	1 cup	389
Evaporated milk, skim	½ cup	371
Collards, cooked	1 cup	357
Ricotta cheese, part skim	½ cup	337
Parmesan cheese	1 oz.	336
Orange juice, calcium fortified	1 cup	333
Milk, skim	1 cup	302
Milk, 1% fat	1 cup	300
Soybean milk, fortified	1 cup	200–300
Soybeans, dry roasted	½ cup	232
Tofu, firm	½ cup	100–200

coach tip

Avoid fish high in mercury. Limit your intake of these fish to once or twice a week or less: swordfish, tuna, king mackerel, shark, and tile fish. If you are breast-feeding or pregnant, do not consume these fish. The greatest danger is to those who are young and growing.

If you do not eat dairy products or want to try a new type of low-fat cheese substitute that melts well, try low-fat or fat-free soy cheeses. These taste quite good and have no dairy fat, so you may want to give them a try. You can find soy cheeses in health-food stores and some supermarkets.

EGGS

Whole eggs are fine to purchase, but if you are watching your fat and cholesterol, remove the yolk before cooking or use egg substitutes. Egg Beaters and Smart Ones make excellent egg substitutes that contain only egg whites with added vitamins and food coloring. Try these if you want to reduce both the fat and cholesterol in your diet. Experiment with the different brands, since each has a distinctive taste.

FISH AND SEAFOOD

Try the many varieties of fresh and seasonal seafood that are now available in supermarkets. If you would like to increase your intake of omega-3 es-

coach tip

The cholesterol in seafood does not affect your cholesterol nearly as much as saturated animal fats do. Therefore, feel free to have shellfish. If you have elevated cholesterol, limit your intake of shellfish to one meal a day.

sential fatty acids, refer to the list of fish that are rich in these fatty acids on page 73 in Step 3. You'll also find a variety of seafood marinades in the fish section of the store. Many of these are delicious and low fat or fat free. If you are watching your sodium intake, check the nutrition labels on the marinades, as some are high in salt. Frozen seafood is a good alternative to fresh, unless it is fried, breaded with butter, or preserved in an oily dressing.

POULTRY AND MEAT

The leanest forms of poultry are chicken, turkey, and Cornish hen—all without the skin. The leanest cut of beef is the round, particularly the eye round and top round. The leanest cut of pork is pork loin. If you want lean chopped meat, ask the butcher to grind the meat from the round or purchase 95 percent lean ground beef.

When you shop for beef, remember that the more white marbling in the beef, the higher its fat content. "Select" beef has the least amount of marbling, followed by "choice," then "prime." Choose "select" beef whenever possible.

THE DELI

Unfortunately, the deli is limited in low-fat choices. Most deli meats are high in fat. The leanest choices of meat at the deli are turkey breast, roast beef with the fat removed, and ham. Roasted chicken is a good choice, but remove the skin before you eat it, since that's where most of the fat is. Healthy Choice and several other companies produce low-fat, prepackaged sandwich meats. Look for them in the meat section.

The prepared meat and fish salads at the deli are usually high in fat because they are mixed with mayonnaise or oil. Avoid these items, or ask the deli manager about the ingredients in any particular salad.

Now that you've toured the perimeter of the supermarket, it is time to begin tackling each of the center aisles. When reading the labels on the prepared foods, please be aware that ingredients are listed on a package by weight, from highest to lowest. For example, if you look at the ingredients list below, you will see that there is more sugar in this product than oil.

Ingredients List: whole-wheat flour, oats, skim milk, sugar, baking soda, vanilla, raisins, salt, oil

If you're watching your salt intake, make sure salt is one of the last ingredients listed on the package. Before you check the ingredients list, refer to the nutrition facts label as a guide. As a rule of thumb, when watching your salt content, use only products that contain 350 mg or less of sodium per serving unless you are further restricted for medical reasons. If the package is labeled "low sodium," it is a sure sign that it is acceptable. Since sodium is found in both natural and packaged foods, try to limit yourself to about 1,500 mg per day of sodium from packaged foods.

BEVERAGES

WATER Bottled sparkling and nonsparkling water can help you meet your daily water allotment. The FDA has several regulations for bottled water. Bottled water must meet the same standards as municipal tap water; water labeled "spring water" must come from a natural spring source; and mineral water that contains a significant amount of calcium, iron, and sodium must list the nutrition contents on the label. Some mineral waters can help you meet your daily requirement for calcium and iron. For example, San Pellegrino's mineral water contains over 200 mg of calcium per liter.

Don't be fooled by the many "imitation water" products, which are clear in color but high in sugar or syrups. Many have the same amount of calories as a piece of fruit but none of the nutritional value. Check the nutrition facts labels on these products carefully.

CAFFEINATED BEVERAGES If you choose to cut down on caffeine, look for decaffeinated beverages, including decaffeinated tea, decaffeinated diet colas, herbal teas to have hot or cold, and cocoa mixes. Be cautious when buying any of the herbal bottled iced teas that are now available: Many are heavily sweetened with honey and thus are high in sugar—so high, in some cases, that they count as a Sweets serving.

BOTTLED JUICES AND DRINKS Bottled lemonade and other natural drinks are better choices than caffeinated beverages. However, they are often flavored with a good deal of sugar, fruit juice concentrate, honey, or corn syrup, which makes them high in sugar. Check the nutrition label: If the fruit drink is not mostly juice, you should consider it a Sweets serving, not a Fruit serving. There are many bottled drinks in the marketplace with added vitamins

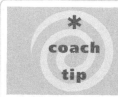

coach tip

BOTTLED WATER — IS IT BETTER?

Not necessarily. You might be surprised to learn that the water from your tap is often just as pure, and sometimes more pure, than the bottled water you can buy. This depends on where you live and the types of pipes that go to your home. If you would like to know about the safety of your water, contact the Environmental Protection Agency (EPA) for more information. The Web site address is www.epa.gov.

and herbs. While I would not give these drinks to children, they are usually safe to drink as an adult. If you are on a prescription medication, please speak to your physician or dietitian before consuming any of these beverages, as they can interfere with your medication. If you are pregnant or breast-feeding, do not consume products with added benefits from herbs.

CEREALS

Look for hot and cold whole-grain cereals. Cereals are a terrific way to meet your daily servings of whole grains. But read the labels carefully. Many are high in fat, sodium, and sugar—exactly what you should avoid. Instead, look for cereal labels that list the grain and not the sugar first. In fact, try to find cereals that list sugar as the fourth or fifth ingredient. A good rule of thumb is to look for cereals that contain no more than 1 gram of sugar for every 5 grams of total carbohydrates. Also look for cereals that are high in fiber. If the nutrition label says the cereal contains 7 or more grams of fiber per serving, it is a high-fiber food. A cereal containing 3 to 6 grams of fiber per serving is a moderate-fiber food. Avoid cereals that contain hydrogenated or partially hydrogenated oil, palm oil, cottonseed oil, or coconut oil. These are all considered "bad" fats.

If you are confused about how much of your favorite cereal is equal to one Active Wellness serving, you can identify the amount of a serving by using the serving size listed on the cereal's nutrition facts label.

BREADS

Make a point of looking for whole-grain breads. Don't be fooled by breads that look brown but aren't whole grain. Check the nutrition label. If the first ingredient listed is not white flour, but whole-wheat flour, oat flour, rice flour, or rye flour, then the bread is probably a whole-grain product. Check the fiber content as well. Bread with 2 grams or more of fiber per serving is an excellent choice.

If you are trying to lose weight, avoid breads that contain dried fruit, which is often high in calories. Remember to follow the low-fat rule to determine which bread products qualify: 3 grams or less of fat per serving. A slice of bread (1 ounce) equals one grain unit on your Active Wellness eating plan.

CRACKERS AND BAKED SNACKS

I am often asked how many crackers or baked snacks equal one grain serving. With the wide variety of crackers and baked snacks available, the serving size on the nutrition label is a reliable guide to how much of an item equals one serving. Also check the nutrition label for fat and sodium content, particularly if you are trying to lose weight or restrict your salt intake. Check the fiber content as well. If they are high fiber, they are probably also whole-grain products.

COOKIES

In the United States, we eat a minimum of eleven pounds of cookies per person per year, and most of those cookies are high in fat and sugar. But there are some exceptions. Look for cookies that have 3 grams or less of total fat per serving, such as graham crackers and gingersnaps. However, keep in mind that fat free does not mean calorie free. Many fat-free cookies are high in sugar. Two cookies usually count as one Sweets serving on your eating plan. Always confirm a serving with the nutrition facts label if you are unsure of how much to eat. Remember, one sweet is equal to up to 120 calories.

BEANS

Beans make great soups and stews. They are also terrific additions to salads, adding color, texture, and fiber. Beans, lentils, and peas—which are also known as legumes—are an excellent source of both low-fat and high-fiber protein. Experiment with the many types of beans in both dried and canned forms. If sodium intake is a concern for you, check the can for the sodium content as it can be quite high. Since most of the sodium is in the canning liquid, rinse the beans well before using them. Lentils and split peas, especially good in soups, are often available only in dried form, but they cook in about twenty minutes.

To reduce the gas in dried beans, cover them with cold water and soak them overnight. Drain them well under running water, then place in a pot and cover with fresh water. Boil the beans until they are tender.

On your eating plan, beans can satisfy *either your protein or grains/starches requirements*. Main-course bean dishes are excellent substitutes for animal protein—½ cup of beans equals about 1 ounce of animal protein.

GRAINS, PASTA, AND RICE

Almost all grains, pasta, and rice make good choices for your eating plan. But be cautious when buying prepackaged frozen and boxed blends of grains, pasta, and rice that contain flavor packets. Many of these flavorings contain ingredients that are high in butter solids and hydrogenated oils. It is helpful to look for preboxed grains when you are trying out new varieties. The box will guide you with cooking and serving directions. Try the many different Middle Eastern, African, and Spanish grains and rice now available at most supermarkets. Each one has its own distinct texture and taste. Whole grains are best if used within a month; otherwise, their natural oils may go rancid. Grains, rice, and pasta all fall into the whole grains/starches group.

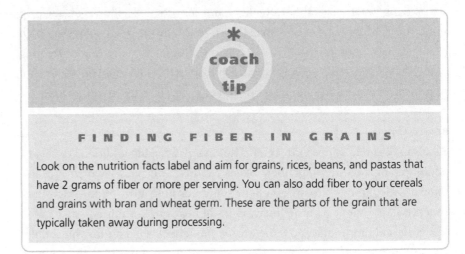

* coach tip

FINDING FIBER IN GRAINS

Look on the nutrition facts label and aim for grains, rices, beans, and pastas that have 2 grams of fiber or more per serving. You can also add fiber to your cereals and grains with bran and wheat germ. These are the parts of the grain that are typically taken away during processing.

SOUPS

Choose from a wide variety of canned, frozen, and freeze-dried soups. All are good choices for your eating plan, since soups are quick and delicious ways to satisfy hunger and fill you up. If you are watching your sodium intake, you may need to avoid many of the freeze-dried soups and some of the canned soups, both of which tend to be high in salt.

Soup can fall into one of three areas in your diet. One cup of vegetable soup or broth is a "free" food. If it is bean soup, it is either a serving from the whole grains/starches group or Proteins group—depending on how you choose to spend your "food servings." If it contains mostly meat and vegetables (for example, stew), do your best to estimate how much meat is in the soup and count it in the Proteins group. The rest of the ingredients are free.

SPREADS AND DIPS

While most Americans use mayonnaise as a spread, it is truly a fat and a saturated one at that. Avoid it whenever possible. The best alternative is using olive oil, or using a soy-based or low-fat mayonnaise, but watch for hydrogenated fats in these products.

Other sandwich spreads, such as mustard and ketchup, are usually fine to use because they are low fat or fat free. But if you are watching your sodium intake or trying to lose weight, check the sugar and sodium content on the nutrition labels. Vegetable and bean spreads are increasingly popular items. They make a wonderful snack when you spread them on low-fat crackers or use them as dips for raw vegetables. You can find them ready-made in most supermarket delis or produce sections or in health-food stores. Guiltless Gourmet makes an excellent bean spread that is sold in many supermarkets. Gourmet vegetable spreads include pumpkin spread, eggplant spread, and roasted red pepper spread. Again, if necessary, check the salt, fat, and sodium content on the label.

SAUCES, SALAD DRESSINGS, AND MARINADES

Check all sauces, salad dressings, and marinades for fat, sodium, and sugar content. A wide variety of these products are available, and their ingredients vary considerably. Follow these rules when buying any of these items:

Total fat per serving should be 3 grams or less
Sodium per serving should be 350 mg or less, if you are watching sodium
for high blood pressure

Tomato sauces and other pasta sauces—except the creamed sauces—are generally healthy alternatives as toppings for pasta, chicken, fish, and even beans. If you like salad dressings, look for those that are low fat and fat free.

FATS AND OILS

Avoid saturated fats, including butter, lard, and hydrogenated vegetable oils such as margarine. If you must use margarine, choose one of the liquid varieties. When buying oils, choose canola oil, olive oil, or peanut oil to use most of the time. These are monounsaturated, the least saturated oils. You can use other seed oils interchangeably, such as sunflower, sesame, or walnut, since seeds and nuts are also unsaturated. Oil usually keeps well in your cupboard for two to four months. Please note that canola oil, the oil that is the most unsaturated, is often made with genetically modified plants. If you have a problem with this ethically, you may want to buy organic.

FROZEN ENTRÉES

Excellent low-fat and vegetarian frozen entrées are available in most supermarkets. Always check their nutrition labels for fat, sodium, and sugar content. Look for low-calorie dinners that derive less than 30 percent of their calories from fat. Frozen dinners are good in a pinch but shouldn't be relied on every day. They are often low in vitamin A, vitamin C, fiber, and calcium. If you eat a lot of frozen dinners, supplement them with fruits, vegetables, and low-fat dairy products to get extra nutrition.

To translate frozen dinner entrées into Active Wellness serving units that satisfy your eating plan requirements, make a best-guess estimate based on how much of the meal, in ounces, is grain, beef, chicken, or fish. If the package lists exchanges, also use these as a guide.

Also check out the frozen-food section for vegetable burgers—low-fat, nutritious, and delicious alternatives to meat for lunch or dinner. Boca Burger, Amy's Organics, Morning Star Farms, and Garden Burger all make excellent veggie burgers in a variety of flavors. You can also find low-fat specialty foods, such as burritos, and a vast array of other international cuisines, including Indian, French, Spanish, and Chinese foods, in the frozen-food section. Be adventurous, but remember to check all of the nutrition labels for fat, sodium, and sugar content.

FROZEN DESSERTS, CAKES, AND PIES

Many frozen desserts, including frozen yogurt and ice cream, sorbet, fresh fruit pops, and ice-cream sandwiches, come in low-fat or no-fat versions.

They make great treats and have the additional advantages of helping curb your appetite and satisfying your sweet tooth.

Low-fat and fat-free cakes are available in frozen and fresh versions. Be cautious when buying these, since many are high in sugar and calories. Check the nutrition label and make sure that low-fat cakes fall within these guidelines:

3 grams or less of fat per serving
120 calories or less per serving
sugar is not the first ingredient listed

Pies are also available in the frozen-food section, but very few offer nutritious choices. Making a good pie is almost impossible without adding a lot of butter to the crust: Even if the filling is sugar free, the crust is probably high in fat. Pie is simply not the best dessert choice for your eating plan.

SNACKS

Snacking is a favorite American pastime. But finding nutritious snacks can be difficult, and determining what makes a healthy portion can be even more difficult. Fortunately, snack foods such as popcorn, tortilla chips, and potato chips now come in low-fat baked varieties. Pretzels are almost always low fat. However, they are also made with processed flours. If you can find whole-wheat pretzels, purchase them instead. For snack foods and pretzels, count the serving size listed on the package as equal to one serving of Grains/Starches on your eating plan.

Nuts, in small quantities, may be eaten as snacks. Be cautious about how many you eat, however, since they are high in fat. Indeed, nuts fall into the Fats category on your eating plan. A serving of nuts is generally six large nuts, like cashews or walnuts, or twenty small nuts, like peanuts, or one tablespoon of seeds. Granola bars and energy bars have become increasingly popular as snack foods, but they invariably are high in sugar and often high in calories. Look for granola and energy bars that are 200 calories or less per serving. If an energy bar is 200 calories, half of the bar counts as one serving of Grains/Starch, assuming the first ingredient is not sugar.

SOY PRODUCTS

Soy products, made from the soybean, are a great source of nutrients and also provide essential fatty acids. Soy products include tofu, tempeh (fermented soy), baked tofu, soy custard, soy protein, soy cheese, soy burgers, and soy nuts, a terrific snack-food item. Many soy products also come in low-fat versions. All the soy products are nutritious alternatives to meat, poultry, and fish. They also help cut down on the saturated animal fats in your diet.

NONDAIRY ALTERNATIVES

If you cannot tolerate cow's milk, try soybean milk or the new rice milks. They both come in a variety of flavors. Several rice milk desserts are available as well.

Setting up your Active Wellness kitchen and restocking your pantry take time, but the dividends are worth it. Below is a shopping list guide with some items you can find at your local store. With delicious, nutritious, and healthful foods close at hand, you're more likely to follow your eating plan and enjoy the process of eating well!

Gayle's Active Wellness Shopping List

This list is designed to help you select healthy foods. Brand names are listed solely for that purpose. Favorite foods of Active Wellness participants were evaluated for inclusion based on the nutritional content information found on the nutrition facts label and the list of ingredients printed on the food packaging. This is not a complete list of healthful foods that meet the Active Wellness guidelines. Inclusion of a food on this list does not imply an endorsement and is not meant to classify any food as "good" or "bad." For foods not on this list, use the Active Wellness guidelines to determine if a food product fits into your personal program.

GRAINS/STARCHES

Bread and bread alternatives; cereals; starchy vegetables; pasta, rice, and other grains; beans; and crackers and snacks

Bread and Bread Alternatives

☐ **Arnold Stoneground**—100% Whole Wheat
☐ **Arrowhead Mills**—Multigrain Pancake and Waffle Mix
☐ **Food for Life**—Certified Organic Grains
☐ **Hodgson Mill**—Organic Pancake Mixes
☐ **Lender's Bagels**—Whole Grain
☐ **Maple Grove Farms of Vermont**—Pancake Mix

- [ ] **Matthew's**—100% Whole Wheat
- [ ] **Mestemacher**—Organic Sunflower Seed Bread
- [ ] **Pepperidge Farm**—Light Style 7 Grain, Very Thin Wheat, Stoneground Whole Wheat
- [ ] **Shiloh Farms**—100% Whole Wheat Hot Dog Buns, and Whole Wheat Bread
- [ ] **Vermont Bread Company**—all

Cereals, Cold and Hot

- [ ] **Arrowhead Mills**—Bulgur Wheat, Multi-Grain Flakes, Oat Bran Flakes
- [ ] **Barbara's Bakery**—100% Natural Shredded Wheat, Multi-Grain Shredded Wheat
- [ ] **Erewhon**—all
- [ ] **General Mills**—Cheerios, Fiber One, Whole Grain Total
- [ ] **Health Valley**—10 Bran, Oat Bran Flakes, Raisin Bran Flakes, Organic Bran
- [ ] **Kashi**—all
- [ ] **Kellogg's**—All Bran, Common Sense Oat Bran, Fruitful Bran, Raisin Bran, Raisin Squares
- [ ] **Mother's**—Oat Bran, Oatmeal
- [ ] **Nabisco**—100% Bran, Shredded Wheat, Shredded Wheat & Bran
- [ ] **Post**—100% Bran, Bran Flakes, Raisin Bran, Shredded Wheat
- [ ] **Quaker**—Instant Oatmeal, Multi-Grain, Oat Bran, Shredded Wheat, Unprocessed Bran
- [ ] **Ralston**—100% Wheat
- [ ] **Wheatena**—Hi Fiber Wheat

Starchy Vegetables

Corn, peas, plantains, potatoes (white, sweet, yams), winter squash (butternut, acorn, etc.)

Pasta, Rice, and Other Grains

All varieties of pasta (unfilled), preferably whole grain, and white, brown, or wild rice, preferably brown or wild varieties
Some brands are:
- [ ] **Azzurro**
- [ ] **Bionaturae Organic Whole Durum Wheat Pasta**
- [ ] **Casbah Pasta and Rice Mixes**
- [ ] **De Boles**

- [ ] **De Cecco Whole Wheat Pasta**
- [ ] **Eden Organic**
- [ ] **Fantastic Pasta and Rice Mixes**
- [ ] **Hodgson Mill Whole Wheat Pasta**
- [ ] **Lundberg**
- [ ] **Marrakesh Express Couscous (fat-free and low-fat varieties)**
- [ ] **Near East**
- [ ] **Papadini Pure Lentil Bean Pasta**
- [ ] **Pritikin Dinner Mixes**
- [ ] **Rice-a-Roni**
- [ ] **Uncle Ben's**
- [ ] **Vita Spelt Organic Whole Grain Pasta**

Beans

Bean soups: see soups (canned or dried, plain)—any
- [ ] **Bearitos**—Lowfat Black Beans, Lowfat Traditional Refried Beans
- [ ] **B&M Baked Beans**—Original, Bacon and Onion, Vegetarian
- [ ] **Bush's Best Baked Beans**—Original Bold & Spicy, Country Style, Onion
- [ ] **Heinz**—Vegetarian Beans
- [ ] **Hormel Chili**—Vegetarian
- [ ] **Old El Paso**—Fat Free Refried Beans, Vegetarian
- [ ] **S&W**—Ranch Barbecue Beans, Maple Sugar Baked Beans
- [ ] **ShariAnn's Organic Refried Beans**—all
- [ ] **Wakim's Foods**—Old Fashioned Hummus, Baba Ganoush

Crackers and Snacks

- [ ] **Ak-mak**—100% Whole Wheat Stone Ground Sesame Cracker
- [ ] **Barbara's Wheatines**
- [ ] **Devonsheer**—Melba Toast, Melba Rounds
- [ ] **Finn Crisp**—Regular, Caraway
- [ ] **Frito Lay Baked Tostitos**—all
- [ ] **Guiltless Gourmet**—all
- [ ] **Herr's**—Baked Bite Size Tortilla Chips, Fat Free Sourdough Bite Size Hard Pretzels
- [ ] **Kame Rice Crunch Crackers**—all
- [ ] **Kavli Crispy Thin**—all
- [ ] **Lavasch Hawaii**—all
- [ ] **Manischewitz**—Whole Wheat Matzos

- [ ] **Mother's Fat Free Rice Cakes**—all
- [ ] **Old London Melba Toast**—all
- [ ] **Quaker Rice Cakes**—Fat Free and Lowfat varieties
- [ ] **Robert's American Gourmet**—Fruity Booty, Nude Food, Pirate's Booty, Power Puffs
- [ ] **Ry-Krisp Natural Crackers**
- [ ] **Ryvita Whole Grain Crispbread**—Dark Rye, Flavorful Fiber, Sesame Rye, Light Rye
- [ ] **Wasa Crispbread**—Light Rye, Sourdough Rye, Multigrain, Hearty Rye, Fiber Rye

VEGETABLES
Canned (no added salt), fresh, frozen (without sauce), tomato sauce, vegetable juice. Avocado and olives—see FATS

Pasta Sauces
- [ ] **Colavita Fat Free**—Marinara, Classic Hot
- [ ] **Millina's Finest Organic Fat Free Pasta Sauce**
- [ ] **Muir Glen Organic**
- [ ] **Pomodoro Fresca**—Original, Ana, Cayenne Hot, Rosemary, Solo

Soups
Look for fat-free or low-fat (less than 3 g of fat per serving) soups. Bean soups are counted as 1 Grain/Starch or 1 Protein serving. Some brands of soup are:
- [ ] **Amy's Organic**
- [ ] **Campbell's Simply Home**
- [ ] **Fantastic**
- [ ] **Hain**
- [ ] **Health Valley Fat Free**
- [ ] **Healthy Choice**
- [ ] **Nile Spice**
- [ ] **Orient Chef Instant Miso Soup**
- [ ] **Pritikin**
- [ ] **Progresso 99% Fat Free**
- [ ] **ShariAnn's Organic**
- [ ] **Tabatchnick**
- [ ] **Walnut Acres Organic Soups**
- [ ] **Woodstock Organics**

PROTEINS
Lean
- [ ] Beans, fish, game (skinless duck breast,

pheasant, goose, rabbit, venison, ostrich, buffalo), lean beef (flank, round, sirloin, top loin, tenderloin, rib/chuck/rump roast, porterhouse/cubed/T-bone steak), lean ham (Canadian bacon), pork loin cuts (tenderloin, center loin, sirloin), skinless poultry (chicken, turkey), shellfish, textured vegetable protein, veal, fat-free or low-fat vegetarian burgers or hot dogs

Egg Substitutes
- [ ] **Better'n Eggs**
- [ ] **Egg Beaters**
- [ ] **Table Ready**

Soy Products (Fat-Free)
Some brands include:
- [ ] **Boca Burger**
- [ ] **Lightlife**
- [ ] **White Wave**
- [ ] **Yves**

Medium Fat
- [ ] **Canadian Bacon**—see FATS
- [ ] **Tofu, tempeh, whole eggs**—for tofu and tempeh, check produce area.
- [ ] **Ocean Beauty**—tuna burger, salmon burger

Soy Products (Low-Fat)
Some brands include:
- [ ] **Boca Burgers**
- [ ] **Gardenburger**
- [ ] **Lightlife**
- [ ] **Morningstar Farms**
- [ ] **Mori-Nu**
- [ ] **Nasoya**
- [ ] **White Wave**
- [ ] **Yves**

THE FRUITS GROUP
(Fresh and frozen fruits, unsweetened fruits canned in water, no sugar-added fruit juices, and dried fruits, unsweetened pureed applesauce varieties)

All fruits, except coconut. See Active Wellness Guidelines for appropriate serving sizes.

DAIRY
Milk and Yogurt
Nonfat or 1% milk (fresh, canned evaporated, and condensed), yogurt, and Lactaid products. Some brands are:
- [ ] **Horizon Organic Fat Free Yogurt**
- [ ] **Silk Cultured Soy Yogurt**
- [ ] **Stonyfield Farm Nonfat and Lowfat Yogurt**
- [ ] **Whole Soy Yogurt**

Rice and Soy Nondairy Beverages
If you are watching your weight, select nonfat or low-fat varieties.
- [ ] **Pacific** (Enriched Rice Delicious Nondairy Drink, Naturally Almond, Select Soy)
- [ ] **Rice Dream**
- [ ] **Vitasoy**
- [ ] **Westbrae** (Natural Rice Beverage, Natural Westsoy)

Cheeses and Sour Cream
- [ ] **Alouette**—Light Spreadable Cheese
- [ ] **Alpine Lace**—Reduced Fat Feta
- [ ] **Athenos**—Reduced Fat Feta
- [ ] **Bonnie Bell Lowfat**
- [ ] **Borden 2% Milk Singles**
- [ ] **Boursin Light Gournay Cheese Spread with Herbs**
- [ ] **Breakstone's**—Fat Free Sour Cream, 2% Lowfat Cottage Cheese
- [ ] **Coach Farm**—Lowfat Goat Cheese
- [ ] **Finlandia**—Heavenly Light 50% Less Fat Swiss
- [ ] **Friendship**—Nonfat Sour Cream, Nonfat and 1% Cottage Cheese varieties
- [ ] **Horizon Lowfat Cottage Cheese**
- [ ] **Jarslberg Lite**—Reduced Fat Swiss
- [ ] **Kraft 2% Milk Singles**
- [ ] **Laughing Cow Lowfat**
- [ ] **Polly-O Lite**—Shredded Reduced Fat Mozzarella
- [ ] **Sargento Lite**—Reduced Fat Shredded Mozzarella

FATS
Oils
Monounsaturated (canola, olive, peanut), polyunsaturated (corn, safflower, sesame, soybean, sunflower, walnut)

Nuts and Seeds
All types, dry roasted or raw, nut butters
- [ ] **Smuckers All-Natural Peanut Butter**

Dressings and Miscellaneous Fats
- [ ] Avocado, bacon (Canadian style), creamers (powder or liquid), low-fat cream cheese, low-fat mayonnaise, low-fat soy mayonnaise, black olives
- [ ] **Annie's**
- [ ] **Blanchard & Blanchard**
- [ ] **Kraft**
- [ ] **Marie's Low Fat**
- [ ] **Wishbone Just 2 Good!**

SWEETS
- [ ] **After Eight Dark Chocolate Thin Mints**
- [ ] **Archway Fat Free Cookies**—Oatmeal, Raspberry, Devil's Food
- [ ] **Gayle's Miracles—the Perfect Chocolate Truffle**
- [ ] **Health Valley**—Fat Free Marshmallow Bars, Fat Free Blueberry Granola Bars
- [ ] **Jelly Beans**
- [ ] **Junior Mints**
- [ ] **Nabisco Fat Free Newtons and Cobblers**—all

Cakes/Pies
- [ ] Angel food cake
- [ ] Lady fingers
- [ ] **Libby's Pumpkin Pie Mix**
- [ ] Shortcake Dessert Shells
- [ ] **Solo Pie Filling**

Frozen Desserts
- [ ] **Ben & Jerry's Lowfat Frozen Yogurt**
- [ ] **Edy's Whole Fruit Sorbet**
- [ ] **Haagen-Dazs Low-fat or Fat-free Frozen Yogurt**
- [ ] **Healthy Choice Low-fat Ice Cream***
- [ ] **Marino's Italian Ices**
- [ ] **Sharon's Sorbet**

Puddings
- [ ] **Imagine Pudding**
- [ ] **Jell-O** (made with skim milk)
- [ ] **Jolly Rancher Gel Snacks**

☐ Kozy Shack Pudding (low-fat)
☐ Swiss Miss Fat Free

Sweeteners
Use sparingly:
Fructose
Honey
Maple syrup
Molasses
Sugar

CONDIMENTS
Cocoa (unsweetened)
Fat-free cream cheese
Fruit jam (naturally sweetened)
Ketchup
Mayonnaise (fat-free, non-fat, or soy based)
Mustard
Oil spray
Salad dressing
☐ **Blanchard & Blanchard Vermont Fat Free**
☐ **Kraft Free**
☐ **Maple Grove Farms of Vermont Fat Free**

Spreads, Sauces, and Miscellaneous
All fat-free or low-fat varieties:
apple butter, barbecue sauce, black bean dip,
chutneys, gravy, lite soy sauce, lite teriyaki sauce,
picante sauce, salsas, taco sauce, Worcestershire
sauce

FROZEN ENTRÉES
Always check the freezer case for new items in this
category.
☐ **Amy's Organic**—Asian Noodle Stir Fry, Bean
   Burritos, Pizzas, Veggie Loaf
☐ **Cascadian Farms** (organic)—Meals for a Small
   Planet
☐ **Cedarlane**—Lowfat Garden Vegetable
   Enchiladas, Lowfat Burritos, Lowfat Veggie
   Wraps
☐ **Hain Vegetarian Classics**
☐ **Healthy Choice***
☐ **Lean Cuisine***
☐ **Thai Chef**
☐ **Veggie Pie Pocket Sandwich**
☐ **Weight Watchers Smart Ones***

WATER EQUIVALENTS
Bouillon, broth, consommé, club soda, herbal
teas, mineral water, unsweetened seltzers,
water

*Some varieties may contain partially hydrogenated vegetable oils and
trans-fats.

Other items _____

_____

_____

_____

_____

Main Points to Putting Your Eating Plan into Practice Anywhere You Are

✔ Your eating plan is designed so you can find foods to eat and feel in control of taking care of yourself around food anywhere you are.

✔ By knowing a few simple strategies, you can ensure that you will not overindulge at restaurants or parties. There is always healthy food to be had.

✔ A key to enjoying your plan is making sure you have a wide selection of foods to choose from. When you use the Active Wellness way of grocery shopping and the shopping list, you will be surprised at how many tasty, healthy foods there are in the marketplace. Have fun and try new things. The more foods you have in your eating repertoire the more enjoyable your eating program.

5

Your Personal Physical Fitness Plan

BY INCORPORATING PHYSICAL activity into your life, you can have an impact on your mind, body, and spirit. This one aspect of your program can increase longevity, help prevent illness and disability, reduce feelings of stress and aging, strengthen physical and mental endurance, and enhance feelings of self-control and self-esteem. Combined with a proper eating plan, physical activity can also boost your energy level, increase your metabolism, and help you efficiently use your nutrients.

The Many Benefits of Exercise

People who exercise regularly get sick less often and experience fewer episodes of depression, anxiety, fatigue, and discouraging emotions. Conversely, a lack of physical activity is associated with diseases such as osteoporosis, heart disease, diabetes, and obesity. The numerous physical, mental, and emotional benefits of exercise are listed in the charts on page 135.

In addition to all the physical, mental, and emotional benefits, regular physical exercise can also aid in slowing down the aging process, helping you to look and feel younger. In fact, the Tufts University Center for Aging has identified ten physical "markers" associated with the aging process, all of which you have the power to modify through physical exercise. They include:

* Lean body mass
* Strength
* Basal Metabolic Rate (BMR)
* Body-fat percentage
* Aerobic capacity
* Blood sugar tolerance
* Total and HDL cholesterol levels
* Blood pressure
* Bone density
* Body temperature regulation

Clearly, exercise is just as important as eating right and is a vital part of your overall wellness program. If you want to lose weight and increase your energy you have to exercise. Although some people think they can accomplish both of these goals through good nutrition alone, a regular physical exercise program, along with proper nutrition, is the only way to permanently increase your energy level and lose weight. It is extremely difficult to succeed in keeping weight off over the years if you don't engage in some type of regular physical activity. In fact, over 90 percent of the people who maintain weight loss have integrated a regular fitness routine into their lifestyles. Therefore, there is no time like the present to think about how you can incorporate physical activity into your weekly health routine!

Overcoming Our Sedentary Natures

The first hurdle we have to face is overcoming an aversion to exercise. Most people average only fifty minutes of regular physical activity a week, when in fact the National Academy of Sciences recently raised the recommendation to sixty minutes of activity a day. The good news is that all activity counts to your sixty minutes, so if you walk up stairs, or walk your dog during the day, you can add that time to your total for the day. Lifting your grandchild or baby on a regular basis, weeding your garden, and mowing your lawn all count as physical exercise. Once you get started with your regular routine, you may find you enjoy physical activity so much, and feel so good, that you'll move on to more challenging exercises.

Overcoming resistance to regular exercise is critical to starting your fitness program, but you'll need to find the initial motivation to get moving within yourself. Our technologically top-heavy lifestyle, dominated by modems, motors, keyboards, and remotes, does not encourage physical activity; in fact, it discourages and even constrains it. Sure, our minds may be racing faster than ever, but our bodies are slowing down. Physical inertia has become the norm, and inertia is a powerful state with a stubborn tendency to perpetuate itself. In addition to this, we have a multitude of excuses for

Physical Benefits of Exercise

Strengthens the Heart
Improves Lung Capacity
Increases Metabolic Rate
Increases Muscle Strength
Improves Cholesterol Levels
Lowers Blood Pressure
Facilitates Digestion
Increases Flexibility and Endurance
Increases Bone Density
Helps Control Blood Sugars
Helps Control Weight
Enhances Immunity

Mental and Emotional Benefits of Exercise

Enhances Self-Esteem
Improves Concentration
Reduces Stress
Promotes Positive Mental Attitude
Promotes Emotional Stability
Increases Mental Energy
Improves Sleep Patterns
Increases Sense of Well-Being
Reduces Negative Emotions
Relieves Anxiety and Tension
Relieves Depression and Fatigue
Improves Quality of Life

why we can't exercise, from disliking sweat to thinking we need a health-club membership to believing we're too out of shape to get started. But by far the most frequent excuse I hear is, "I just don't have the time to exercise." Ironically, the truth is that once you make time for exercise, exercise will create more time in your life. You'll need less sleep, have more energy, work more efficiently, and become more productive; all of which make more free time to do the things you enjoy the most. If you are willing to hurdle the inertia barrier and make time for regular physical fitness in your life, I promise tremendous physical, mental, and spiritual payoffs.

coach
tip

General Signs of Exercise Intolerance

If any of the symptoms listed here occur during or after exercise, consult your doctor or go to your nearest medical facility as soon as possible.

• Pain or pressure in the chest, arm, or throat during or immediately after exercise. If this does occur, go to the nearest emergency room. These may be signs of a heart attack.
• Substantial increase in shortness of breath with exercise.
• Dizziness, light-headedness, sudden lack of coordination, confusion, or fainting.
• Sudden burst of rapid heartbeats or sudden slowing of a rapid pulse.
• Nausea or vomiting.

Beginning Your Fitness Program

As with your eating plan, your physical fitness plan is unique to your own needs, interests, and abilities. As you begin to put the components of your program together, it is essential to follow these two guidelines:

① Start slowly, particularly if you have been leading a sedentary lifestyle or have specific health concerns.

② Be realistic about what you can initially accomplish at your current level of fitness.

The following Health History Questionnaire and Physical Fitness Questionnaire will help you follow these guidelines. Answering the questions on both forms will help you determine which exercise plan is right for you.

Health History Questionnaire

		Yes	No
1	Do you now have, or have you ever had, a history of heart problems, chest pain, or stroke?	——	——
2	Do you now have, or have you ever had, high blood pressure?	——	——
3	Do you now have, or have you ever had, high blood cholesterol?	——	——
4	Do you now have, or have you ever had, any chronic illness or condition?	——	——
5	Do you now have, or have you ever had, difficulty doing physical exercise?	——	——
6	Have you ever been advised by a physician not to exercise?	——	——
7	Have you had surgery within the last 12 months?	——	——
8	Are you now pregnant, or have you been pregnant within the last 3 months?	——	——
9	Do you now have, or have you ever had, a history of breathing or lung problems?	——	——
10	Do you have any muscle, joint, or back disorders?	——	——
11	Do you have diabetes or a thyroid condition?	——	——
12	Do you smoke or have you smoked within the last year?	——	——
13	Are you currently overweight (more than 20 percent above your ideal weight)?	——	——
14	Are you 40 years of age or older?	——	——

If you answered "yes" to any of the above questions, you should consult your physician before beginning this or any exercise program. Certain clinical conditions, including diabetes, heart disease, and metabolic disorders, require advice from a physician before initiating any exercise program. And while individuals at any age can begin moderate exercise programs, men over age forty and women over age fifty who plan to start an exercise program should consult a physician first. Whether or not you need to consult your doctor, you can design your fitness program now, then show it to him or her before you begin.

Your Current Physical Fitness Level

Next you need to determine your current level of physical fitness, regardless of any current or past medical conditions. The following fitness assessment questionnaire will help you put together a realistic, safe, and gratifying exercise program that will be tailored to your current physical capabilities.

Physical Fitness Questionnaire

OCCUPATION AND DAILY ACTIVITIES

1 I walk at least one-half mile on most days (e.g., to and from work or my shopping area). _____ (1 point)

2 I usually take stairs rather than using elevators or escalators. _____ (1 point)

3 The type of physical activity involved in my job or daily household routine is best described by the following statement:

    a. Most of my workday is spent doing office work, light physical activity, or household chores. _____ (0 points)

    b. Most of my workday is spent doing moderate physical activities, brisk walking, or comparable activities. _____ (4 points)

    c. My typical workday includes several hours of heavy physical activity (shoveling, lifting, etc.). _____ (9 points)

LEISURE ACTIVITIES

1 I do several hours of gardening or yard work each week. _____ (1 point)

2 I fish or hunt once a week or more. (Fishing must involve rowing a boat; sitting on the dock does not count.) _____ (1 point)

3　At least once a week, I participate for an hour or more in vigorous dancing, such as square or Latin dancing (or another activity that requires continual movement). _____ (1 point)

4　I play golf at least once a week without using a golf cart. _____ (1 point)

5　I often walk for exercise or recreation. _____ (1 point)

6　When I feel bothered at work or at home, I use exercise as a way to relax. _____ (1 point)

7　Two or more times a week I perform calisthenic exercises, such as sit-ups and push-ups, for at least 10 minutes per session. _____ (3 points)

8　I regularly do yoga or stretching exercises. _____ (2 points)

9　I participate in active recreational sports such as tennis or handball:
  a. Once a week _____ (2 points)
  b. Twice a week _____ (4 points)
  c. Three or more times a week _____ (7 points)

10　I participate in vigorous fitness activities such as jogging, swimming, aerobic exercises, or cycling for at least 20 continuous minutes per session:
  a. Once a week _____ (2 points)
  b. Twice a week _____ (4 points)
  c. Three or more times a week _____ (7 points)

TOTAL SCORE: _____ POINTS

Review the chart below to determine your current physical fitness level.

Your Current Physical Fitness Level		
Score	**Activity Level**	**Effect on Fitness**
0–5 points	Sedentary	This amount of exercise is insufficient and leads to a steady decrease in fitness. Improvement is needed.
6–11 points	Light	This amount of exercise increases fitness somewhat but will not maintain adequate fitness levels in most persons.
12–20 points	Moderate	This amount of exercise maintains an acceptable level of physical fitness.
20+ points	Active/Very Active	This amount of exercise maintains an active superior level of physical fitness.

The Physical Fitness Chart

Activity Level (Intensity)	Activities	Calorie Expenditure (Men)	Calorie Expenditure (Women)
Sedentary	Lying; resting; sitting; sitting while performing light desk work	1 calorie/min.	1 calorie/min.
Light	Bowling; fishing; golfing; horseback riding; strolling; vacuuming; stationary light cycling; standing while performing light work	2–5 calories/min.	2–4 calories/min.
Moderate	Dancing; fast walking; hiking; light swimming; pleasure cycling; racquet sports; leisurely roller skating/Rollerblading	5–8 calories/min.	4–6 calories/min.
Active	Aerobic dance; basketball; canoeing; jogging; walking uphill with weights; fast cycling; fast swimming; downhill and cross-country skiing; touch football; competitive racquet sports; roller skating/Rollerblading	8–10 calories/min.	6–8 calories/min.
Very Active	Fast-paced jogging; cycling; downhill and cross-country skiing; speed walking; swimming; basketball; football; racquet sports; mountain climbing; roller skating/Rollerblading; wrestling	10–13 calories/min.	8–10 calories/min.

Comparing the Different Activity Levels

The Physical Fitness Chart above will give you a better idea of the types of exercises that are included in each activity level: "sedentary," "light," "moderate," "active," and "very active." You can also see approximately how many calories you burn per minute at each level. There are more calories burned per minute at a higher level of activity, because these exercises require more effort.

However, if you are trying to burn calories for weight loss or to maintain your weight, it is less strenuous on the body to burn calories by exercising for longer periods of time at a lower intensity or low impact. Low-impact exercises also help reduce your risk for injury and are easier to sustain for a longer duration. Fast walking at moderate intensity is an excellent example of an exercise that is low impact. The more you walk, the more calories you burn and the more fit you become. Take a minute while you are reviewing

Food Equivalents of Common Exercises

Food Type	Approximate Calorie Count	Light Intensity*	Moderate Intensity**	Active/Very Active Intensity***
Breakfast				
1 large bagel with 2 tbsp. cream cheese	500	2 hr. 47 min.	1 hr. 23 min.	1 hr. 3 min.
1 3-oz. muffin	300	1 hr. 40 min.	50 min.	38 min.
1 8-oz. low-fat yogurt	220	1 hr. 13 min.	37 min.	28 min.
1 cup cereal with ½ cup nonfat milk	155	52 min.	26 min.	19 min.
1 slice of bread	80	27 min.	13 min.	10 min.
Lunch/Dinner				
1 slice of pizza with cheese	350	1hr. 45 min.	1 hr.	45 min.
1 hamburger, medium, single patty	280	1 hr. 33 min.	47 min.	35 min.
4 oz. cooked pasta	140	47 min.	23 min.	18 min.
1 cup of lentil soup	140	47 min.	23 min.	18 min.
1 3-oz. chicken breast	130	43 min.	22 min.	16 min.
Snacks/Dessert				
1 piece pie (⅛ of 9-inch pie)	300	1 hr. 40 min.	50 min.	38 min.
1 2-oz. brownie	270	1 hr. 30 min.	45 min.	34 min.
1 oz. mixed nuts, dry roasted	170	57 min.	28 min.	21 min.
1 1-oz. bag of potato chips	150	50 min.	25 min.	19 min.
1 chocolate chip cookie	140	47 min.	23 min.	18 min.
1 oz. tortilla chips	140	47 min.	23 min.	18 min.
½ cup vanilla ice cream	130	43 min.	22 min.	16 min.
½ cup frozen yogurt	115	38 min.	19 min.	14 min.
1 oz. pretzels (small bag)	110	37 min.	18 min.	14 min.
1 medium apple or banana	100	33 min.	17 min.	13 min.
1 cup cooked vegetables	100	33 min.	17 min.	13 min.
Alcohol				
1 5-oz. glass of wine	100	33 min.	17 min.	13 min.

Calorie expenditures calculated as the average of calorie expenditures for men and women.
*Light Intensity Activity expends approximately 3 calories per minute, on average, and includes: bowling; fishing; golfing; horseback riding; strolling; vacuuming; stationary light cycling; standing while performing light work.
** Moderate Intensity Activity expends approximately 6 calories per minute, on average, and includes: dancing; fast walking; hiking; light swimming; pleasure cycling; racquet sports; leisurely roller skating/Rollerblading.
***Active/Very Active Intensity Activity expends approximately 8 calories per minute, on average, and includes: aerobic dance; basketball; canoeing; jogging; walking uphill with weights; fast cycling; fast swimming; downhill and cross-country skiing; touch football; competitive racquet sports; roller skating/Rollerblading.

the chart to estimate how many calories you burn throughout the week. Include walking to and from your car as well as your routine exercise. A goal for weight loss is to use 300 to 500 calories in energy for activity each day. This will help you burn your excess storage fuel (fat), so you become leaner.

How Much Energy Does Your Body Burn?

Food is packed with energy. So, it is easy to eat more than our bodies need and more than we can burn in exercise. The Food Equivalents chart on page 141 will give you an idea of how to equate your energy burn in exercise to foods you may be eating.

Designing Your Personal Fitness Plan

In your fitness plan, you will be choosing activities that match your current fitness level. As you determine the activities you want to incorporate into your life on a weekly basis, I will ask you to periodically take time to enter your information into the Personalized Exercise Program (P.E.P.) Worksheet on page 170. You can use the P.E.P. Worksheet to help you organize your weekly fitness goals.

The best fitness programs are those that are *consistent,* because consistency at the appropriate intensity can increase your level of fitness gradually while minimizing injury. You can use the recommendations of the American College of Sports Medicine (see the box on page 143 and Coach Tip on page 147) to establish your personal fitness goals as you move forward in planning your personal weekly exercise routine.

Your Five Fitness Plan Essentials

The five basic activities that comprise your total weekly exercise program will include: (1) warm-ups, (2) aerobic/cardiovascular workout, (3) muscle toning/strength training, (4) stretching exercises, and (5) cooldowns.

1. WARM-UPS

Warm-ups are essential because they prepare your body for the more rigorous demands of the aerobic and strength-training exercises that will follow. When your body is at rest prior to beginning your workout, your muscles are receiving only a small percentage of the blood that is circulating throughout your body. Warming up increases bloodflow to the muscles, which literally "warms" them. This makes the muscles more pliable and flexible, which helps protect your body against unnecessary injuries and muscle soreness. Warm-ups also allow your body's temperature to adjust gradually to the increased bloodflow that occurs during a more vigorous exercise.

Warm-ups should be done for ten minutes prior to exercise. Many times your warm-up routine can consist of the same type of activity that you do for your aerobic exercise, just at a slower or more leisurely pace. Walking and low-intensity cycling are great warm-up exercises. They target most of the major muscle groups, allowing you to begin slowly and to ease into your workout. At the end of your warm-up, your body will be well primed for your aerobic or strength-training activities.

Take a moment to record your warm-up routine on your P.E.P. Worksheet. Refer to the Physical Fitness Chart on page 140 to choose your warm-up activity. The warm-up exercise you choose should be at an intensity level that is one level lower than your current fitness level. For example, if you exercise at a moderate intensity, you will begin your warm-up at a light intensity. Only if you are at a light-intensity level should your warm-up be the same as your current activity level.

2. AEROBIC/CARDIOVASCULAR WORKOUT

The word *aerobic* means "with oxygen." Aerobic fitness refers to the ability of your heart and lungs to effectively deliver oxygen-carrying blood to large groups of working muscles during sustained and continuous physical movement. Aerobic exercise, properly done, utilizes oxygen to improve the fitness of your heart and lungs. Your heart is a muscle, and one of the best ways to keep it in shape is to exercise it with aerobic activities that strengthen the heart muscle just as they strengthen the other muscles of the body.

Aerobic activity is a great way to burn fat. When a large supply of oxygen reaches your body's cells, your body burns fat more effectively by using the fat as energy to fuel the muscles. This fat-burning ability increases as the duration of your aerobic exercise increases and your level of fitness improves. It takes approximately twenty minutes of continuous exercise before fat is available as a fuel source for your body. The more fit you are and the longer you exercise, the more calories and fat you will burn.

For those of you who are just beginning a fitness program and cannot

coach tip

The American College of Sports Medicine has kept its recommendation for aerobic activity to: Exercise three to five days a week at moderate intensity for thirty to forty-five minutes, despite the sixty minutes recommended by the National Academy of Science. Better to just get moving, according to its view, by aiming for thirty minutes per day and working up to sixty minutes. The general consensus is the more fit you are the healthier you are.

begin exercising at a high level of intensity, rest assured you can also burn calories and fat during low-intensity exercises, like walking, which is a huge step in the right direction along the path to wellness.

The best aerobic exercises utilize the large muscle groups of the body (the legs, buttocks, chest, and arm muscles) and involve continuous and repetitive movements without a lot of stopping and starting. Some of the more popular and challenging aerobic activities are included in the list below.

Common Aerobic Activities

Brisk Walking/Jogging	Dancing
Spinning Classes	Continuous Rope Skipping
Rowing	Rollerblading
Biking	Swimming
Cross-Country Skiing	Stairmaster Workout
Roller Skating/Ice Skating	Hiking
Step Aerobics	Stairclimbing

FINDING YOUR PERSONAL INTENSITY LEVEL FOR AEROBIC ACTIVITY Exercise intensity is measured in two ways. One is how fast your heart beats during an activity. The other is how difficult you perceive the activity to be. To determine how fast your heart should beat during aerobic activity, you need to know your maximum heart rate (MHR) and your target heart rate (THR). Your maximum heart rate (MHR) is the maximum number of times your heart can physiologically beat per minute during exercise. It is the threshold point for your heart, beyond which it becomes too difficult for your body to exercise and you will be forced to stop. Your target heart rate gives you a goal of how many beats per minute your heart should beat during aerobic activity.

It is best to exercise at a percentage of your maximum heart rate, or target heart rate. Research shows that the best way to achieve fitness is to perform aerobic activities with a target heart rate (THR) range. Your THR range is 60 to 80 percent of your maximum heart rate. To determine your target heart rate you can use the equation below. Or, if you have had a stress test or a thorough fitness test within the last month, you were probably given your MHR and THR at that time. No one should exercise at their maximum heart rate (MHR).

Maximum heart rate
MHR = 220 − your age

Target heart rate
MHR × .60 = _____
This is the lower number of your THR range, measured in beats per
    minute.

THR = MHR × .80 = _____
This is the upper number of your THR range, measured in beats per
    minute.

For example, if you are forty years old, your maximum heart rate is 220 − 40 = 180 beats per minute. Your THR at forty years old would be 180 × .60 = 108, which is the minimum number of beats per minute you want to achieve when you are performing aerobic activity. No one should exercise at their maximum heart rate (MHR). If you have a heart condition or are on blood pressure medication, your heart rate may be lower than these calculations. Consult your physician before determining your THR range.

Determine your maximum heart rate and target heart rate now, and record it on your P.E.P. Worksheet (page 170).

HOW TO MEASURE YOUR TARGET HEART RATE It is important to know how to measure your heart rate while you are exercising so that you can be sure that you're within your target heart rate range during your aerobic workout. You can do this by locating your pulse and counting your heartbeats. After you have warmed up and have been exercising aerobically for five minutes, lightly place your index and middle fingers on the side of your neck below your jawbone, or on the inside of your wrist. When you feel a steady pulse,

*
coach
tip

If you are highly active, you can adjust the upper limit of your target heart rate to take into account your higher fitness ability. Do this by multiplying the upper range by .85 (85 percent) instead of .80 (80 percent).

count the number of beats (or pulses) for six seconds. Multiply this number by ten to get your heart rate, or count a total of sixty seconds of heart beats. This number should fall within your target heart rate range. If it is lower

Testimonial

I started Active Wellness because I needed to do something to get healthier, drop weight, and improve my high risk for heart disease. I didn't want to go back to my cardiologist and have him up my medication again. It was time for me to take action. I liked Active Wellness right away, because I am the type of person who just needs to be told what to do and I can execute it.

I first addressed my eating. Since I dine out a lot for business, I needed to learn how to manage the amount of food and wine I was consuming so that I didn't eat more than my body needed. Just changing my eating plan helped me drop about twelve pounds. Then, I began to revamp my exercise routine. With the guidance from Active Wellness I was able to create a total exercise approach that covered aerobic, strength training, and stretching. I realized that lifting weights was not really helping to strengthen my heart, so I added aerobic exercises and gradually worked up to an "Active" activity level through cycling and jogging. Exercise and feeling fit really give me a sense of accomplishment and gratification. Since I exercise in the morning before work, I know I have done something good for myself everyday, and that feels good. Once I had my exercise program in place I added a stress-management routine to my program. I am very pleased with my results. My cholesterol profile has greatly improved, my HDL has gone way up, I am now taking half my cholesterol medication, my blood pressure is under control, and I have lost over twenty pounds. I have a new lease on life. I feel younger than I have felt in years!

While there were many programs to choose out there, I've always felt that it is important to learn from a professional, and this program really helps you to succeed, because you take it at your own pace. I know I can continue to live the Active Wellness way, because I made it my own, and I feel so good, I don't want to go back to my old ways.

Larry, age fifty-six, weight loss 22 pounds, lowered cholesterol, reduced medication, reduced heart-disease risk

than your THR range you may need to increase the intensity of your activity and speed up. If the number is above your THR range, you are working out too hard and may need to decrease your intensity and slow down. You can also use a heart-rate monitor to check your target heart rate. They can be found at stores that sell running and biking equipment.

THE FINE ART OF PACING-CHALLENGING YOURSELF You are the best judge of your fitness level and how to pace yourself with your aerobic conditioning. Always keep in mind that if you try to do too much too soon, you can damage your body by injuring your muscles or overexerting your heart, raising your heart rate to levels that are not conducive to a quality aerobic workout. Therefore, remember to increase your physical fitness gradually, by pushing yourself only slightly beyond your comfort zone. Your workout or activity should always feel somewhat challenging, but never painful or unduly uncomfortable.

When you feel comfortable at your current level of exercise, challenge yourself by pushing, just a bit more beyond that plateau. In this way, you continually increase your cardiovascular fitness, muscle strength, and stamina to your optimal capacity. Three aerobic diagram charts are provided below that will help you to pace yourself. Start with the chart that best matches your activity level—light, moderate, or high—and record your weekly plan for aerobic exercise on your P.E.P. Worksheet. You can use the Sample Fitness Calendar on page 169 as a guide.

CHOOSING YOUR AEROBIC PLAN The activity levels for aerobic activity are listed in order of difficulty. Choose the level that best matches your needs and ability. Plan your first week of activity based on the charts provided and record your weekly plan on your P.E.P. Worksheet.

SEDENTARY OR LIGHT ACTIVITY GUIDELINES If you have been sedentary or fairly inactive, don't worry about reaching your target heart rate when you first start your exercise program. Begin your program with physical activities that increase your heart rate slightly but do not feel strenuous or exhausting. Light-intensity activities include such things as leisurely walking, taking the stairs, yard work, housework, gardening, or light biking.

For the first two weeks of your fitness program, do twenty to thirty minutes of light physical activity three to five days per week. Thereafter, add five

American College of Sports Medicine Exercise says you can achieve the most benefits from exercise when you reach and maintain your target heart rate at a goal of 60 to 80 percent of your maximum heart rate during twenty to sixty minutes of exercise, three to five days per week.

minutes a day to your routine each week until you have reached a goal of fifty to sixty minutes of light physical activity at least five days a week. You may also do a combination of varying short-term activities that add up to your fifty- to sixty-minute total per day.

As you progress each week, your endurance and stamina will increase. You will gradually move up to the next level of exercise, where you can achieve a new level of maximum aerobic benefit.

Aerobic Program—Light Activity			
Week	Warm Up	Aerobic Activity Aiming To Reach Your Target Heart Rate (Exercise Time) Activities = walking, light biking, walking up stairs.	Frequency (Days/Week)
1–2	10 minutes (walking or walking up stairs)	10 minutes week one 15 minutes week two	3 days/week
3–4	10 minutes (walking or walking up stairs)	20 minutes week three 25 minutes week four	3 days/week
5–6	10 minutes (walking or walking up stairs)	30 minutes week five 35 minutes week six	4 days/week
7–8	10 minutes (walking or walking up stairs)	40 minutes week seven 45 minutes week eight	4 days/week
9–10	10 minutes (walking or walking up stairs)	50 minutes week nine 60 minutes week ten	5 days/week
11–12	10 minutes (walking or walking up stairs)	60 minutes week; then increase distance (pick up your pace, but stay within target heart rate)	5 days/week
13–14	10 minutes (walking or walking up stairs)	60 minutes week; then increase distance (pick up your pace, but stay within target heart rate)	5 days/week
15–16	10 minutes (walking or walking up stairs)	60 minutes week; then increase distance (pick up your pace, but stay within target heart rate)	5 days/week

*Remember, you can break up your exercise time into shorter sessions that total the recommended time allotment.

MODERATE ACTIVITY GUIDELINES Exercises that fall into the moderate-intensity category include brisk walking, jogging at an easy pace, moderate aerobics, cycling at a medium pace, swimming, hiking, and cross-country skiing at a leisurely pace. At this level you should be exercising at your target heart rate range.

Start your moderate exercise routine with ten minutes of warm-up exercises. During the first two weeks of your program, try to do twenty to thirty minutes of moderately intense aerobic exercise three or four days a week. After two weeks, add five minutes a day to your aerobic routine each week until you reach a maximum of fifty to sixty minutes, which may be broken into two twenty-five- or thirty-minute sessions a day. Once you can comfortably maintain this level of exercise, gradually increase the frequency of your workouts to four or five days a week. At this stage, you have reached a healthy level of fitness, and, depending on the personal fitness goals you have established, you can either maintain your aerobic routine or move on to higher-intensity activities.

ACTIVE/VERY ACTIVE ACTIVITY GUIDELINES Exercises that fall into the high-intensity category include jogging, swimming, heavy aerobics, cross-country skiing, and cycling—all performed at a rapid pace. If you are just beginning to exercise at the active level, you'll want to gradually incorporate the higher-intensity exercises into your routine, without changing the number of days per week you exercise. Begin your aerobic routine with a ten-minute warm-up, followed by your aerobic activity, then a five- to ten-minute cooldown. For the first two weeks, perform your aerobic exercise for fifteen to twenty minutes, three or four days a week. Then, every two weeks, begin adding five minutes a day to your routine until you reach a maximum of forty-five to fifty minutes a day of intense aerobic activity. Once you are able to exercise at this level, you can increase your exercise sessions to five days a week. Or, you can choose to maintain your aerobic sessions to four days a week and focus on using the remainder of the week for strength training and stretching, the other fitness components that will complete your exercise routine.

Take a moment to make sure you have entered all your aerobic information on the P.E.P. Worksheet. Also, select the days in your week that you are planning to schedule time to accomplish your warm-up and aerobic exer-

Aerobic Program—Moderate Activity

Week	Warm Up 10 minutes (e.g., walking, light jogging in place, cycling)	Aerobic Activity at Your Target Heart Rate Duration (Exercise Time) Activities = brisk walking, cycling, beginner-intermediate aerobic classes.*	Cool Down with light aerobic activity (e.g., brisk walking) and stretching	Frequency (Days/Week)
1–2	10 minutes	20–30 minutes/day	5 min. lower intensity aerobic 5 min. stretching	3–4 days/ week
3–4	10 minutes	25–35 minutes/day	5 min. lower intensity aerobic 5 min. stretching	3–4 days/ week
5–6	10 minutes	35–40 minutes/day	5 min. lower intensity aerobic 5 min. stretching	4–5 days/ week
7–8	10 minutes	45–50 minutes/day	5 min. lower intensity aerobic 5 min. stretching	4–5 days/ week
9–10	10 minutes	50–60 minutes/day	5 min. lower intensity aerobic 5 min. stretching	4–5 days/ week
11–12	10 minutes	60 minutes week; then increase distance (pick up pace, but stay within target heart rate) or increase time by 5–10 min.	5 min. lower intensity aerobic 5 min. stretching	4–5 days/ week
13–14	10 minutes	60 minutes week; then increase distance (pick up pace, but stay within target heart rate) or increase time by 5–10 min.	5 min. lower intensity aerobic 5 min. stretching	4–5 days/ week
15–16	10 minutes	60 minutes week; then increase distance (pick up pace, but stay within target heart rate) or increase time by 5–10 min.	5 min. lower intensity aerobic 5 min. stretching	4–5 days/ week

*Remember, you can break up your exercise time into two sessions.

cises. As you progress, you can change your P.E.P. Worksheet to reflect your new routine.

Once you have your aerobic routine worked out, you can begin to incorporate weekly muscle toning/strength training and stretching exercises.

Aerobic Program—High Activity

Week	Warm Up 10 minutes (e.g., walking, light jogging in place, cycling)	Aerobic Activity at Your Target Heart Rate Duration (Exercise Time) Activities = brisk jogging, cycling, beginner-intermediate aerobic classes.*	Cool Down with light aerobic activity (e.g., brisk walking) and stretching	Frequency (Days/Week)
1–2	10 minutes	15–20 minutes/day	5 min. lower intensity aerobic 5 min. stretching	3–4 days/ week
3–4	10 minutes	25–30 minutes/day	5 min. lower intensity aerobic 5 min. stretching	3–4 days/ week
5–6	10 minutes	35–40 minutes/day	5 min. lower intensity aerobic 5 min. stretching	4–5 days/ week
7–8	10 minutes	45–50 minutes/day	5 min. lower intensity aerobic 5 min. stretching	4–5 days/ week
9–10	10 minutes	55–60 minutes/day	5 min. lower intensity aerobic 5 min. stretching	4–5 days/ week
11–12	10 minutes	60 minutes week; then increase distance (pick up pace, but stay within target heart rate) or increase time by 5–10 min.	5 min. lower intensity aerobic 5 min. stretching	4–5 days/ week
13–14	10 minutes	60 minutes week; then increase distance (pick up pace, but stay within target heart rate) or increase time by 5–10 min.	5 min. lower intensity aerobic 5 min. stretching	4–5 days/ week
15–16	10 minutes	60 minutes week; then increase distance (pick up pace, but stay within target heart rate) or increase time by 5–10 min.	5 min. lower intensity aerobic 5 min. stretching	4–5 days/ week

*Remember, you can break up your exercise time into two sessions.

3. MUSCLE TONING/STRENGTH TRAINING

Strength-training activities strengthen and tone muscles through weight or resistance exercises. Strength-training workouts can be performed using free weights, resistance bands and tubing, or your own body weight as resistance. In strength training, you exercise with progressively heavier weights or in-

coach tip

FINDING YOUR COMFORT ZONE: PERCEPTION OF EXERCISE DIFFICULTY

Regardless of your calculated fitness level, you have to "listen" to your body while you are exercising. You should never experience any sensation of physical straining. You should always feel able to complete your exercises comfortably, within the recommended time frame and without having to stop and rest.

A good rule of thumb is to make sure you can say a full sentence while you are exercising without gasping for air. If you can't, your body is not receiving enough oxygen and you could injure yourself.

creased resistance to develop physical endurance and increase the strength of your muscles and skeletal system. This training can have a profound effect on your physical strength and your appearance by increasing your lean muscle mass. As we get older, it is the extra muscle mass that helps us maintain our weight, because muscle burns more than fat, a greater muscle mass means your body needs more energy to function each day and you can eat more because of it.

Both men and women can increase their muscle mass by about three pounds by following a ten-week strength-training program. Strength training also slows the aging process, improves posture and balance, and increases energy and stamina. The Active Wellness strength-training program is provided in this section. However, I strongly advise that you see an exercise specialist before you begin strength training to ensure that your posture and positioning are correct when you work out. Exercise specialists are available at most health clubs and YMC/HAs, or you can hire a personal trainer to come to your home. It is worth the investment in time and money to work with a trainer once or twice before starting out on your own. He or she can observe your form, make modifications to your program, and help protect you against any long-term damage. Alternatively, you can rent or buy a strength-training video to work out with or take a strength-training class.

THE COMPONENTS OF YOUR STRENGTH-TRAINING PROGRAM The key to performing strength-training exercises properly is using progressive resistance (weights) to build muscle. Schedule your strength-training exercises at least two days per week. It is best to have a day between your strength-training workouts to give your muscles a chance to relax. As with your aerobic exercise routine, you should warm up and cool down before any strength-training exercises.

After completing your warm-up, do 8 to 12 repetitions (known as a set) of each of the eleven exercises (pictured on pages 155 to 159) that are designed to condition all the major muscle groups. If you can't do a minimum of 8 repetitions of each exercise, you probably are using too much resistance or weight. If this is the case, decrease the weight or resistance until you can comfortably do 8 to 12 repetitions. If you are just beginning, do not use weights or resistance bands for your first session. See how you feel just by using your own weight as resistance and follow the movements indicated in the program.

Unless you perform regular muscle-toning exercises, you will lose up to a half-pound of muscle every year of your life after the age of twenty-five!

If you are just starting out, you will not need weights for the strength-training exercises. However if you feel you can lift the weight of your arms easily, then it is recommended that you invest in light weights, either 3 or 5 pounds, or resistance bands. Both Dynabands and Xertubes are inexpensive resistance bands that provide the same weight resistance as free weights. The Xertubes have the additional advantage of having handles, which makes them easier to grip. Both bands come with their own instruction book and set of resistance exercises and are available in most sports equipment and department stores.

You may also want to purchase an exercise ball. Exercise balls are a lot of fun. Aside from the two exercises included in the strength-training routine, the exercise ball should also come with diagrams of additional exercises.

Also remember to work all the muscle groups, so that no one muscle group becomes stronger than another. For instance, if you do sit-ups to strengthen your stomach muscles, remember to strengthen your back muscles as well; otherwise your stomach muscles can pull your body out of alignment from an imbalance of muscle strength. Review the strength-training workout on the following pages and enter your strength-training program on your P.E.P. worksheet, designating days of the week for your strength-training routine.

Aim to perform two to three sets of 8 to 12 repetitions of each exercise, giving yourself a thirty- to sixty-second rest between each set. Each set should be done in a slow, controlled fashion that allows you to maintain your breath throughout the exercises. When you can perform three sets of an exercise comfortably and with good form, try varying your set patterns, your tempo, and the different muscle groups you focus on. Once you can complete two or three sets comfortably, you can increase the weight/resistance you are using (by approximately 5 percent) to continue to increase muscle strength.

General Strength-Training Program—Light Activity

Week	Weight/Resistance	Repetitions	Frequency (Days/Week)
1–2	No weight or resistance	5–10 repetitions of each exercise without strain.	1–2 sessions/week
3–4	No weight or resistance	8–12 repetitions of each exercise without strain.	2 sessions/week
5–6	Light weight or light resistance	8–12 repetitions of each exercise without strain.	2 sessions/week
7–8	Light weight or light resistance	5–10 repetitions of each exercise without strain. Increase to two sets of 8–12 repetitions of each exercise.	2 sessions/week
9–10	Increase resistance by 5 percent if you are achieving your current resistance level with ease	5–10 repetitions of each exercise without strain. Increase to two sets of 8–12 repetitions of each exercise.	2–3 sessions/week

Resistance Note: Do not increase resistance until you are achieving the recommended number of repetitions comfortably. Also, remember to breathe during each exercise.

Repetition Note: The goal is to achieve 10–12 repetitions of each exercise per set. If you are working toward this goal, begin with the number of repetitions you can complete comfortably without strain and increase this number by 2 repetitions each week until you reach the goal of 12 repetitions for each exercise.

General Strength-Training Program—Moderate Activity

Week	Weight/Resistance	Repetitions	Frequency (Days/Week)
1–2	Light weight or light resistance	8–12 repetitions of each exercise without strain.	1–2 sessions/week
3–4	Light weight or light resistance	8–12 repetitions of each exercise without strain. Increase to two to three sets of 8–12 repetitions of each exercise.	2 sessions/week
5–6	Light weight or light resistance	8–12 repetitions of each exercise without strain Increase to two to three sets of 8–12 repetitions of each exercise.	2 sessions/week
7–8	Increase resistance by 5 percent if you are achieving your current resistance level with ease	8–12 repetitions of each exercise without strain. Increase to two to three sets of 8–12 repetitions of each exercise.	2 sessions/week
9–10	Maintain resistance level from week 8	8–12 repetitions of each exercise without strain. Increase to two to three sets of 8–12 repetitions of each exercise.	2–3 sessions/week

Resistance Note: Do not increase resistance until you are achieving the recommended number of repetitions comfortably. Also, remember to breathe during each exercise.

Repetition Note: The goal is to achieve 10–12 repetitions of each exercise per set. If you are working toward this goal, begin with the number of repetitions you can complete comfortably without strain and increase this number by 2 repetitions each week until you reach the goal of 12 repetitions for each exercise. Increase the number of sets up to three per exercise; when you achieve this comfortably, increase resistance by 5 percent.

1. Lunge: Standing with feet shoulder-width apart, step forward with one leg. Hold your head, shoulders, and chest high and look forward. Bend your front leg to a right angle, making sure your knee is in line with your ankle, while bending your other knee without allowing it to touch the floor. Repeat 10 to 12 times on the same leg. Switch legs and repeat. (Light hand weights are optional.) *Breathing:* Exhale as you lunge, inhale as you return to the starting position.

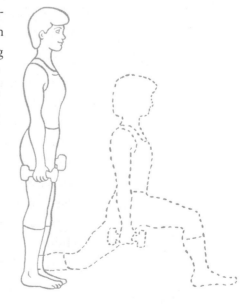

General Strength-Training Program—High Activity

Week	Weight/Resistance	Repetitions	Frequency (Days/Week)
1–2	Adequate weight or resistance to achieve 8–12 repetitions with some effort, but no strain	10–12 repetitions of each exercise without strain. Two sets.	3 sessions/week
3–4	Maintain weight/resistance level during week 2	10–12 repetitions of each exercise without strain. Two sets.	3 sessions/week
5–6	Increase resistance by 5 percent if you are achieving your current resistance level with ease	10–12 repetitions of each exercise without strain. Two sets.	3 sessions/week
7–8	Maintain weight/resistance level during week 6	10–12 repetitions of each exercise without strain. Two sets.	3 sessions/week
9–10	Increase resistance by 5 percent if you are achieving your current resistance level with ease	10–12 repetitions of each exercise without strain. Two sets.	3 sessions/week

Resistance Note: Do not increase resistance until you are achieving the recommended number of repetitions comfortably. Also, remember to breathe during each exercise.

Repetition Note: The goal is to achieve 10–12 repetitions of each exercise per set. If you are working toward this goal, begin with the number of repetitions you can complete comfortably without strain and increase this number by 2 repetitions each week until you reach the goal of 12 repetitions for each exercise. Increase the number of sets up to three per exercise; when you achieve this comfortably, increase resistance by 5 percent.

2. Side Leg Lift: Begin from a standing position with your feet together, hands holding on to a wall or chair. Raise one leg to the side, making sure you're standing straight. Keep your hipbones forward and straight and keep the raised leg straight with toes slightly turned inward, throughout the exercise. The supporting leg should be slightly bent. Lift your leg up and down 10 to 12 times and then repeat with the other leg. *Breathing:* Inhale when you lift your leg, exhale when you bring it back to meet your supporting leg.

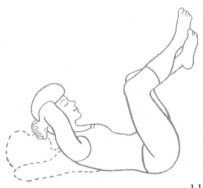

3. Leg Lift: Sit tall with your back straight and chest lifted. You can sit against the wall for support if that helps you. Place your legs straight out in front of you. Bend one leg, placing your foot flat on the floor. Lift your other leg 5 to 8 inches from the floor, then slowly lower it to about an inch off the floor and repeat. Keep your foot and knee pointed upward throughout the exercise. Repeat 10 to 12 times. Switch to the other leg to complete the sequence.
Breathing: Exhale as you lift, inhale when you bring your leg down.

4. Abdominal Curl: Lying on your back with your hands behind your head, cross your feet and bring them up, keeping your lower back on the floor. Keep your knees over your abdomen. (If you prefer, you can keep your feet on the floor with your knees bent.) Lift your head and neck up to the base of your shoulder blades using your stomach muscles, then return to the starting position. Do not strain your neck, use your hands as a support. Repeat 10 to 12 times. *Breathing:* Inhale as you lift up, exhale as you return to the starting position.

5. Prone Head and Leg Lift: Lie down on your abdomen with your arms bent and your palms on the floor, hands facing forward by your shoulders. Begin with your chin on the floor. Slowly lift your head and one leg off the floor, lifting your leg from your hip. Repeat this exercise with one leg at a time; repeat each leg 10 to 12 times. *Breathing:* Exhale as you lift, inhale when you return to the starting position.

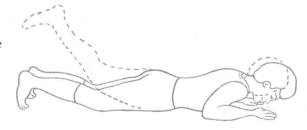

6. Push-ups: Lying on your abdomen, push your body up with your hands, keeping your back straight from your knees to your head. Keep your neck in line with your spine. Contract your abdomen. Repeat push-ups 10 to 12 times or as many as you can accomplish.

Breathing: Exhale as you push up, inhale when you come down.

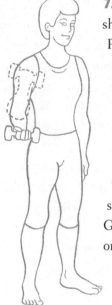

7. Biceps Curls (with weights): Stand tall with feet shoulder-width apart. Grip the weight with one hand. Place your elbow close to your body, with your palm facing upward. Curl your arm up slowly. Pause and return to the starting position. Repeat with each arm 10 to 12 times to complete the sequence. *Breathing:* Exhale as you lift, inhale as you lower.

8. Side Lateral Raises (with weights): Stand with your feet shoulder-width apart. Grip the weight with one hand, with your palms facing your body. Raise your arm sideways, up and away from the side of your body, until you reach just below your shoulder. Pause and slowly return to the starting position. Repeat 10 to 12 times with each arm to complete one sequence. *Breathing:* Exhale as you lift, inhale as you lower.

9. Triceps Press Down (with weights): Stand up straight. Place a weight in each hand making sure your arms are parallel to the floor and facing inward. Stand straight. With your arms bent at a 90-degree angle, lower both arms so that they face the floor. As you lower your arms, rotate your hands so your palm faces behind you when your arms are straight; pause and bring your arms back to the starting position, slowly. Repeat with each arm 10 to 12 times to complete the sequence. *Breathing*: Exhale as you lower, inhale as you lift.

THE HIDDEN BONUS OF STRENGTH TRAINING By combining both aerobic exercise, which burns fat, with resistance/weight training, which increases muscle, you can burn more fat and increase your muscle, or lean body mass, which is the ratio of fat to muscle throughout your body. In fact, focusing on reducing "fat mass" and increasing "lean mass" may be a better fitness focus than setting a weight goal. Fitness trainers and medical technicians have elaborate methods for determining the ratio of lean muscle mass to fat mass, including the skinfold assessment test, underwater (hydrostatic) weighing, and the bioelectric impedence technique. If you can avail yourself of one of these assessment measures, by all means do so. While these measurements can be helpful, you should be able to see the results of your efforts (a decrease in fat mass and an increase in muscle mass) just by looking at your body and noticing the way your clothes fit.

4. STRETCHING EXERCISES

Stretching exercises are the best way to improve and maintain your body's flexibility and balance. Many people neglect this component of physical fitness because they don't realize the importance of improving the range of physical motion (flexibility) and maintaining the suppleness of muscles, joints, and connective tissue. Stretching exercises enhance your fitness routines by making it easier and safer to move, bend, and lift without injury and fatigue. Stretching also helps relieve stress by releasing muscle tension.

When holding your stretch, don't bounce; aim for a sustained, comfortable stretch. Also, remember yoga can count as a stretch routine and a stress-management routine.

   If you are flexible, start at your current level and aim for a goal to increase your frequency (days/week) or duration(minutes/session).

Stretching, or flexibility, exercises were once thought of as warm-ups, or what you did before you started your "real" exercise workout. This is definitely no longer the case. In fact, you need to warm up before you do any stretching/flexibility routines. You can take stretching or flexibility classes at many gyms, health clubs, and YMC/Has. Other physical activities, such as ballet, yoga, and t'ai chi, are also considered stretching exercises. I recommend that you do formal stretching exercises for thirty to sixty minutes at least twice a week. However, when stretching is done correctly, it is very gentle on the body and can be done every day. It is a great idea to add ten minutes of stretching exercises after you have completed your aerobic and strength-training workouts, since your muscles will already be warmed up, more flexible, and primed for stretching. The important fact to remember about stretching is that you should never force a stretch or try to bounce up and down to achieve a stretch. The correct way to stretch is to aim for a sustained and comfortable stretch without straining, and with your attention focused on the muscle you are working on. Forcing a stretch can activate the "stretch reflex," where a signal is sent to the muscle to shorten and contract to keep it from being injured. Ironically, if you stretch too far, you will actually tighten the muscles you are trying to stretch and lengthen.

When you are stretching correctly, you should feel mild tension as the muscles and connective tissue elongate. This should not be painful and the tension should decrease as you hold the stretch for ten to twenty seconds. After ten to twenty seconds, ease off slightly and find a lesser degree of tension within your comfort zone. Hold this stretch for another ten to thirty seconds. The goal here is no pain and great gain. An illustrated stretching routine follows. Take a moment now to record the dates and time of your stretching program on your P.E.P Worksheet (page 170).

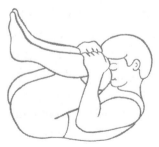

1. For your back: Lie on your back on the floor. Bring both legs toward your chest, as shown in the diagram. Curl your head toward your knees and hug your legs to your chest. Hold for 10 seconds; when you release this stretch, straighten out both legs so they are lying on the floor and bring your hands and head

General Stretching Program—All Flexibility Levels

Week	Warm Up (at your current intensity level)	Duration (Time) of Stretch	Repetitions	Frequency in Days/Week and Minutes/Day
1–2	10 minutes	20 seconds/stretch	2–5 repetitions/exercise	1–2 sessions/week 15–30 minutes/day
3–4	10 minutes	20 seconds/stretch	2–5 repetitions/exercise	1–2 sessions/week 15–30 minutes/day
5–6	10 minutes	20 seconds/stretch	2–5 repetitions/exercise	2 sessions/week 20–40 minutes/day
7–8	10 minutes	20 seconds/stretch	2–5 repetitions/exercise	2 sessions/week 25–45 minutes/day
9–10	10 minutes	20 seconds/stretch	2–5 repetitions/exercise	3 sessions/week 30–60 minutes/day

Repetition Note: See specific exercises in Stretching Exercises in this chapter to guide you with the number of repetitions for each movement. When holding the stretch, do not bounce; aim for a sustained comfortable stretch. Also, remember yoga can count as a stretch routine and a stress-management routine. If you are very flexible, start at your current level and aim for a goal to increase your frequency (days/week) or duration (minutes/session). Remember, stretching can be done every day without harming your body.

back to rest on the floor. Repeat this stretch 3 times, or as many times as it feels good to you.

2. **For your lower back and hips:** Lying on the floor, place both arms to your sides. Bend one knee to a 90-degree angle (see diagram) over the other leg that is straight. Turn your head in the direction opposite your bent leg. Using the arm that is on the same side as the bent leg, pull your bent leg down toward the floor until you feel a comfortable stretch in your lower back and hip. Do not force a stretch if it is painful. Hold this 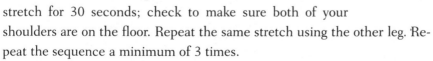 stretch for 30 seconds; check to make sure both of your shoulders are on the floor. Repeat the same stretch using the other leg. Repeat the sequence a minimum of 3 times.

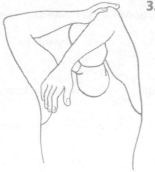

3. For shoulders, arms, and upper back: Stand with feet shoulder-width apart. Place one arm behind your head. Hold the bent arm with your free arm (see diagram). Gently pull down on your bent elbow until you feel a stretch. Repeat this with your other arm. Hold the stretch for 15 seconds. Repeat the sequence a minimum of 3 times.

4. For legs and hips: Sit on the floor on your knees. Place one leg forward, bending at the knee, so that your knee is in line with your ankle. Rest your other knee on the floor with your back leg and foot out behind you (see diagram). Holding this position, shift your weight forward so that you move your hip downward until you feel a stretch. The movement should be gentle. When you feel the stretch, hold this position for 30 seconds. Repeat with your other leg in front. Repeat the sequence a minimum of 3 times.

5. For groin and hamstrings: Sitting on the floor, place the soles of your feet together, as close together as they can go. Holding your feet, pull forward from your hips—not your back—until you feel a stretch. Hold this position for 40 seconds or less if you feel pain. Release. Repeat 3 times at a minimum. Be careful not to bounce when you are in this position.

6. For back, shoulders, and arms: Start from a kneeling position. Lean forward and stretch your arms as far out as you can, keeping arms staight. Gently press down on the floor with the palms of your hands. Hold this position for 30 seconds. Do not bounce. Return to a kneeling position. Repeat the sequence a minimum of 3 times.

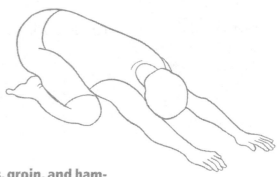

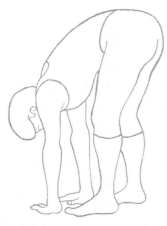

7. For lower back, hips, groin, and hamstrings: From a standing position, bend your knees slightly and then bend forward from your waist—hanging your arms over your head and let your head go, with your crown facing the ground. Reach as far to the floor as you can. Hold this position for 30 seconds. Do not bounce. Return to a standing position. Keep your knees slightly bent and repeat the sequence a minimum of 3 times.

5. COOLDOWNS

The final component of your physical fitness program is cooldowns. These are as vital to your program as warm-ups, aerobic, strengthening, and stretching exercises. Cooldowns allow the cardiovascular system to gradually return to its normal levels. This stage is especially important if you have a risk of heart disease, are older, or are just starting to allow the heart rate to safely decrease to 120 beats per minute or less. It also prevents blood from pooling in the lower extremities, where it can cause reduced blood pressure, dizziness, and, in some rare cases, cardiac arrhythmias.

You can use a slower-pace aerobic exercise to cool down, such as walking, slow cycling, or slow Stairmaster. Whatever exercise you choose, the important aspect during cooldown is to watch your heart rate to make sure it slowly comes down. Perform cooldown exercises for ten to fifteen minutes at a decreasingly slower pace. Cooling down will help decrease possible muscle soreness and stiffness.

How to Challenge Yourself

You can increase your physical endurance during exercise in three ways:

* By increasing the frequency of the exercise (how often you do it)
* By increasing the intensity of the exercise (how hard you do it)
* By increasing the duration of the exercise (how long you do it)

It is very helpful to understand how to integrate the above components of frequency, intensity, and duration into your plan. The best way to raise your fitness level is to focus on increasing just one of the above components at a time. For instance, if you walk thirty minutes a day (duration), three to five days a week (frequency), on flat terrain (intensity), you may want to increase the duration of your activity after two weeks. Start walking thirty-five minutes a day, three to five days a week on the same terrain.

What you don't want to do is increase your duration at the same time you increase the intensity of the walk (by changing to an uphill terrain, for example) or the frequency of the walk (by adding an extra day to your regimen). You may tire out too soon or get injured, leaving you more discouraged than motivated.

Sometimes people who have been sedentary for a long time suddenly decide to get in shape and start exercising intensely every day. By the end of the first week, every muscle in their body aches and they have to stop exercising to give their body time to heal. This can start a self-defeating cycle of stop-and-start exercising. Once you stop a routine, even briefly, you may have a hard time getting motivated to start again. I cannot emphasize enough that at the outset of your fitness program you should establish reasonable and realistic goals for yourself and begin exercising gradually and moderately as you increase your ability.

Strategies for Success Away from Home

How many times have you gone off your health regimen because you went on a vacation or business trip? Not being in your usual environment makes it more challenging to remain on your new healthy routine. Traveling for work or pleasure can become an easy justification for letting go of your self-

Testimonial

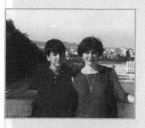

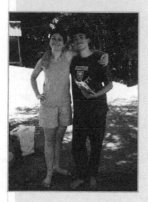

A year ago, at forty-nine years old, I was thirty pounds overweight. I hadn't exercised in years and I got exhausted just climbing the stairs out of the subway. With two kids and a full-time job, I had decided that life was hard enough without worrying about how I looked. But somehow, turning fifty like that was just too depressing. For six months I woke up every morning deciding to start my diet—but by lunchtime it was all forgotten.

Then, by total luck, I heard about Active Wellness. The first week, I was inspired by Gayle's approach. The program didn't seem like a diet—more like a philosophy about feeling good and doing good things for yourself. I could get enthusiastic about that! I decided to make my goal to hike up a mountain for my fiftieth birthday. I figured if I could do that, then I wouldn't feel like I was getting older. I began following the eating plan and I lost my first pound. I stuck to my eating program, even though I was losing weight slowly at first, because I felt so good. I began walking to work. I felt even better, and patience paid off. I began losing two pounds every week. By my birthday, I had nearly lost the whole thirty pounds. I felt so good, I dyed my hair red and bought new clothes—even a new bathing suit, which I hadn't done since my son was born seventeen years ago, and I went hiking for my birthday!

I kept going, and a few weeks after my birthday, I reached my goal weight! A year later, Active Wellness remains a very positive part of my life. I never did go on a "diet." I fell in love with yoga and find a few minutes for it every morning. At fifty, I look better, I feel better, and best of all, I'm truly younger than I was before. If Active Wellness could get me going, I know it will inspire you to find the positive, slimmer you!

Laurie, lost 30 pounds and found balance, health, and youth at age fifty

control. Then, when you return home, you may have difficulty resuming your health routine.

Before you know it, three weeks have gone by and you haven't been able to get your eating, exercise, and stress management under control. Beware! The "off the program" blues can really get you down, which can be discouraging. You may feel like you have to begin at the starting line all over again. Luckily, this doesn't have to be the case.

In this step you'll learn strategies for maintaining your Active Wellness Program away from home, whether you are dining out for just one evening or traveling on vacation for several weeks. You will learn how to make your Active Wellness Program "portable" and carry it with you into many different environments. You will also learn how to plan ahead to deal with obstacles along your wellness path, so that being away from home becomes an easier transition for you.

PHYSICAL FITNESS AWAY FROM HOME

Exercising away from home is fairly simple these days because many hotels have fitness centers on-site. Also, many fitness centers allow you to use their facilities for a day if you're away from home. Easy-to-pack fitness accessories allow you to exercise right in your hotel room. But wherever you go, bring along your sneakers and workout attire. If there is a pool, bringing your swimsuit is also a good idea!

MAKING FITNESS EASY

If no gym is available, be prepared to adapt your program to your environment by locating a place to walk or jog and using some easy-to-pack fitness tools. In fact, you can liven up your daily walk or jog by taking a mini "walking tour" through your new surroundings. All three components of your physical fitness program—stretching, aerobics, and strength training—can be adapted for practice away from home.

STRETCHING AWAY FROM HOME In general, a stretching routine can be done anywhere, providing you have a small space in your room. If your room doesn't have enough space, try stretching outside your room in the hallway, or outdoors in the sunshine when the weather is good. If you do your stretching routine in the morning, you'll feel more alert throughout the day. Once you stretch, move on to the aerobic or strength-training portion of your program.

AEROBICS AWAY FROM HOME If you can't find a gym in the area where you are staying, adapt your aerobic program to the environment you are in. One of the easiest ways to do aerobics is to walk at a brisk pace, which can be done just about anywhere. Brisk walking for twenty minutes quickly burns approximately 100 calories—the equivalent of jogging for ten minutes.

If you normally jog, this is an easily transportable activity, as long as you remember to pack your sneakers and make sure you don't get lost in an unfamiliar neighborhood. You may also want to pack a portable radio and headphones, so that you can listen to music while you're walking or jogging. An upbeat tempo will also help you keep up your pace.

If you're traveling strictly on business, your time is more limited than if you are traveling for pleasure. Nevertheless, you may find time for one or more of the following activities: walking; jogging; going to a gym; playing racquetball, tennis, or golf (briskly walking the course); and swimming.

If you're on vacation and traveling simply for pleasure, you can choose from a number of aerobic activities. These might include cycling, Rollerblading, ice skating, row boating, hiking, and water skiing. You can rent the necessary equipment in most larger cities and towns.

STRENGTH TRAINING AWAY FROM HOME Lugging weights around in your suitcase is not a practical way to travel. You can, however, keep up with your strength training on the road by using your own weight as resistance or by bringing along resistance bands for working out.

Replacing Your Old Exercise Shoes

When deciding whether to purchase new exercise shoes before you start your exercise program or along the way, consider this: If you have tendonitis, heel pain, leg pain, blisters, calluses, or pain in the balls of your feet, your shoes are no longer providing adequate support. You also should check your exercise shoes for structural wear and tear, including whether the rubber in the heel has narrowed, the cushioning has diminished, or the shoes bend inward or outward.

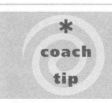

coach tip

Replace running and walking shoes after every 300 to 500 miles of use. Replace aerobic and tennis shoes after every 150 to 200 hours of use.

If you notice when you walk or jog that you are placing more emphasis on the inside or outside edge of your foot, you may want to try orthotics, which can help you balance all your energy on the correct portions of you foot. Orthotics are supports for your feet that are made of either hard plastic or leather. You can insert them into your shoes for additional support. If you think you need orthotics, I recommend that you see an orthopedist to be fitted appropriately.

Types of Exercise Shoes and Their Features

Walking shoes: Forefoot flexibility and cushioning
Running shoes: Cushioning, heel counter, and traction
Aerobic shoes: forefront flex grooves, cushioning, and lateral support
Cross-training: lateral support, cushioning, and traction
basketball: lateral support, cushioning, heel and forefoot cushioning
Tennis: lateral support, durability, traction, and cushioning

Main Points to Your Personal Fitness Plan

✔ Exercise is a critical component of your Active Wellness Program. It affects your energy, immune system, stress level, and longevity.

✔ It is important to determine what level of fitness you are at now, so that you can organize an exercise routine to match your ability. Exercise is not enjoyable when you engage in activities that are too difficult.

✔ Exercise should be fun, so choose activities you like.

✔ There are three components to a well-rounded fitness plan: aerobic exercise, strength training, and stretching. Each discipline tones a different part of your body: Aerobic tones your heart and lungs, strength training tones your muscles, and stretching helps you keep your flexibility.

✔ Active Wellness provides you with actual strength training and stretching routines along with guidelines for including aerobic exercise and personalizing a total program that can work for you anywhere you are.

Sample Fitness Calendar—Starter Plan for Light–Moderate Activity Level

Sunday	Monday	Tuesday	Wednesday	Thursday	Friday	Saturday
Walk 20–30 min. Check Target Heart Rate.	Strength Training 8–12 repetitions of each exercise with light weights (3–5 lbs.) or exercise bands.	Walk 20–30 min. Check Target Heart Rate.	Stretch Program (p. 158 in book) or try Pilates, Ballet, or Yoga tapes/classes.	Walk 20–30 min. Check Target Heart Rate.	Strength Training 8–12 repetitions of each exercise with light weights (3–5 lbs.) or exercise bands.	Walk 20–30 min. Check Target Heart Rate.
Aerobic 20–30 min. (Walk, bike, try the Stepper or other aerobic activity.) Check Target Heart Rate.	Strength Training 8–12 repetitions of each exercise with light weights (3–5 lbs.) or exercise bands.	Aerobic 20–30 min. (Walk, bike, try the Stepper or other aerobic activity.) Check Target Heart Rate.	Stretch Program (p. 158 in book) or try Pilates, Ballet, or Yoga tapes/classes.	Aerobic 20–30 min. (Walk, bike, try the Stepper or other aerobic activity.) Check Target Heart Rate.	Strength Training 8–12 repetitions of each exercise with light weights (3–5 lbs.) or exercise bands.	Walk 20–30 min. Or try biking, the Stepper or other aerobic activity. Check Target Heart Rate.
Aerobic 25–35 min. (Walk, bike, try the Stepper or other aerobic activity.) Check Target Heart Rate. ALSO, Stretch (see Wednesdays).	Strength Training 8–12 repetitions of each exercise—two sets—with light weights (3–5 lbs.) or exercise bands.	Aerobic 25–35 min. (Walk, bike, try the Stepper or other aerobic activity.) Check Target Heart Rate.	Stretch Program (p. 158 in book) or try Pilates, Ballet, or Yoga tapes/classes.	Aerobic 25–35 min. (Walk, bike, try the Stepper or other aerobic activity.) Check Target Heart Rate.	Strength Training 8–12 repetitions of each exercise—two sets—with light weights (3–5 lbs.) or exercise bands.	Aerobic 25–35 min. (Walk, bike, try the Stepper or other aerobic activity.) Check Target Heart Rate.
Aerobic 25–35 min. (Walk, bike, try the Stepper or other aerobic activity.) Check Target Heart Rate. ALSO, Stretch (see Wednesdays).	Strength Training 8–10 repetitions of each exercise with light weights (3–5 lbs.) or exercise bands.	Aerobic 25–35 min. (Walk, bike, try the Stepper or other aerobic activity.) Check Target Heart Rate.	Stretch Program (p. 158 in book) or try Pilates, Ballet, or Yoga tapes/classes.	Aerobic 25–35 min. (Walk, bike, try the Stepper or other aerobic activity.) Check Target Heart Rate.	Strength Training 8–12 repetitions of each exercise with light weights (3–5 lbs.) or exercise bands.	Aerobic 25–35 min. (Walk, bike, try the Stepper or other aerobic activity.) Check Target Heart Rate.
Aerobic 35–40 min. (Walk, bike, try the Stepper or other aerobic activity.) Check Target Heart Rate. ALSO, Stretch (see Wednesdays).	Strength Training 10 repetitions of each exercise with light weights (3–5 lbs.) or exercise bands.	Aerobic 35–40 min. (Walk, bike, try the Stepper or other aerobic activity.) Check Target Heart Rate. ALSO, Stretch (see Wednesdays).				

Personalized Exercise Program Worksheet (P.E.P. Worksheet)

Current Activity Level: _____   Goal Activity Level: _____

Initial Fitness Goal: _____

Target Heart Rate Range: _____

Selected Aerobic Activities: _____

Maximum Heart Rate: _____

Days of the Week	Warm-Ups (check off the days you do aerobic activities)	Aerobic Routine		Strength-Training Routine	Stretching Routine	Cool Down/ Cool-Down Stretching (check off the days you do aerobic activities)
		Aerobic Activity	Exercise Time			
Monday						
Tuesday						
Wednesday						
Thursday						
Friday						
Saturday						
Sunday						

Ways to Manage Stress

YOU JUST MISSED your exit on the freeway. Someone in the car behind you is honking his horn. You have a deadline at work. The house is a mess. You have a cold. The bills are higher than usual this month. You have to race to catch your train. You spend the day worried about a loved one. Or you're expecting a baby. You're getting married. You're training for a marathon. Your youngest child is going off to college. You just got a big promotion. Big or small, happy or sad, unexpected or routine, any of the events just described can trigger stress in your body, mind, and spirit. You can't see, hear, or smell stress, but eventually you feel it—as anxiety, exhaustion, moodiness, sleep disturbances, headaches, shortness of breath, a racing heart, or a stiff neck, to name just a few of its symptoms.

Although we cannot control what stresses us, we can learn how to respond to stress so that it does not affect us negatively. Since all change, including positive change, causes some degree of stress, stress is an unavoidable part of our lives. The symptoms of stress can impact on all aspects of our lives, including eating patterns, digestion, mood, sleep, energy, and immunity to disease. While not all stress is bad—in fact, some stress is necessary for us to function and survive—adverse stress can take a terrible toll on overall health.

In this step we focus on managing our adaptive responses to the type of stress that has a negative impact on us physically, mentally, or emotionally. Learning how to respond to negative stress will help you bring balance to your life. You'll learn a variety of techniques and coping skills to help you combat the effects of stress and integrate stress management as a permanent part of your Active Wellness Program.

Defining Stress

Stress is difficult to define or even recognize, because stress means different things to different people. What you regard as stressful, another person might find invigorating or challenging. For example, a job loss may plunge one individual into feelings of worthlessness and depression. Another person might see a job loss as a chance to reshape his or her career and move on to more interesting and rewarding work.

Our responses to what we perceive as stressful are unique; they are our physical, emotional, and psychological responses to a situation, event, or stimulus. Often stress is perceived as threatening or challenging to our personal well-being, family, loved ones, finances, work, or social standing.

Determining Your Stress Index

The physical and emotional damage caused by stress can make us miserable, but, oddly enough, we often aren't even aware that we are under stress. The signs and symptoms of stress, together with the habits and attitudes we adopt to cope with it, are so familiar and commonplace to us that we simply accept them as part and parcel of our lives. How high is your stress index? Find out by completing the brief questionnaire on page 173.

Long-Term Effects of Stress

Stress Response	Long-Term Effect(s)
Storage energy mobilized for use by muscles	Eventual fatigue; no excess energy available for storage
Elevated triglycerides, fats, and glucose (sugar) in the blood	Increased risk for elevated triglycerides, cholesterol, and diabetes (for those at risk)
Increase in blood pressure	Greater chance of forming plaque in arteries and developing chronic hypertension
System shutdown of digestion	Peptic ulcer; indigestion
Other system shutdowns (reproductive; tissue building)	Lack of ability to reproduce; loss of libido; decalcification of bones
Depression of immune response	Decreased disease resistance

Stress Index Questionnaire

Do you frequently: Yes   No

1 Neglect your diet?   ___   ___
2 Try to do everything yourself?   ___   ___
3 Blow up easily?   ___   ___
4 Seek unrealistic goals?   ___   ___
5 Fail to see the humor in situations that others find funny? ___   ___
6 Act rude?   ___   ___
7 Make a "big deal" of everything?   ___   ___
8 Look to other people to make things happen?   ___   ___
9 Complain that you are disorganized?   ___   ___
10 Avoid people whose ideas are different from yours?   ___   ___
11 Keep your emotions inside?   ___   ___
12 Neglect exercise?   ___   ___

13 Have few supportive relationships?   ___ ___
14 Use sleeping pills and tranquilizers without a
    doctor's approval?   ___ ___
15 Get too little rest?   ___ ___
16 Get angry when you are kept waiting?   ___ ___
17 Ignore stress symptoms?   ___ ___
18 Put things off until later?   ___ ___
19 Think there is only one right way to do something? ___ ___
20 Fail to build relaxation time into your day? ___ ___
21 Gossip?   ___ ___
22 Race through the day?   ___ ___
23 Spend a lot of time complaining about the past? ___ ___
24 Fail to get a break from noise and crowds?   ___ ___

Total your score: Count 1 for each "yes" answer
and 0 for each "no" answer.

YOUR SCORE: ____

Adapted from the Stress Index, courtesy of Canadian Mental Health Association, Saskatchewan Division.

What Your Score Means:

1–6: There are few hassles in your life. Make sure, though, that you are not trying so hard to avoid problems that you are also shying away from challenges.

7–13: You've got your life under fairly good control. Work on the choices and habits that may still be causing some unnecessary stress in your life. The suggestions in this chapter should help.

14–20: You're approaching the danger zone. You may well be suffering stress-related symptoms, and your relationships could be strained. Think carefully about choices you've made and take relaxation breaks every day.

Read this chapter carefully and follow the suggestions to better manage your life.

Above 20: Emergency! You must stop now, rethink how you are living, change your attitudes, and pay careful attention to diet, exercise, and relaxation. There are many suggestions in this chapter that can help you live a healthier, happier life.

Although the effects of stress in our daily lives may seem unavoidable, we can learn many techniques to offset the damage done by stress. For one thing, take a look at how you personally respond to stress and then make conscious choices about changing your stress-coping methods. You can also use any of the techniques described in this chapter to enjoy the benefits of healthful stress management.

What Are Your Stressors?

The situations, events, or stimuli that trigger a stress response are called "stressors," and they fall into the following three main categories.

CATACLYSMIC STRESSORS

Cataclysmic stressors include natural or man-made disasters such as hurricanes, earthquakes, fires, and tornadoes. While they can be devastating events that cause acute stress in the short term, they occur infrequently.

BACKGROUND STRESSORS

Background stressors include "environmental" stressors of a repetitive or routine nature that we feel we cannot control. They include, among other things, a neighbor's barking dog or blaring music; long commutes and traffic jams; a high-pressure career or a monotonous, dreary job; and constant background noise at work or at home. Because they are part of our daily lives and not always easy to recognize or acknowledge, background stressors are potentially very damaging, gradually gnawing away at our sense of well-being.

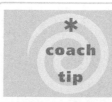

coach tip

Ask yourself how you can create less stress in your life. What will it take? Make a list of what you feel you need to do and then narrow it down to three things you want to take action on. Then make a commitment to complete your list within a specific time frame.

PERSONAL STRESSORS

Personal stressors include threatening or challenging situations, events, or stimuli that impact on us in a highly personal manner. They might include the death of a loved one; having a baby; the loss of a job; the breakup of a marriage; buying a home; personal injury or illness; a major career move; nursing an ill parent or spouse; or coping with an abusive spouse or boss. Personal stressors often demand the most from us in terms of coping and adapting, which makes them particularly detrimental to our physical and emotional health.

Personal stressors are usually broken down into five distinct types, but a great deal of overlap occurs among the types. Further, what starts out as one type of personal stressor may rapidly evolve into another. Retirement, for example, is an emotional stressor that may eventually evolve into an intellectual stressor.

THE FIVE TYPES OF PERSONAL STRESSORS

Physical stressors. Anything that causes physical discomfort or forces the body to continually adapt or cope is a physical stressor. Chronic pain and sudden or chronic illness are examples of physical stressors.

Emotional stressors. Significant life events such as a divorce, death of a loved one, loss of a job, retirement, or empty-nest syndrome are emotional stressors. Emotional stress often leads to anxiety, depression, moodiness, and poor physical health.

Intellectual stressors. Common short-term, intellectual stressors include giving a major speech; taking final exams; or facing a complex problem that requires sharp, rational thinking when one simply is not up to it, for instance, doing one's income taxes. It is also intellectually stressful when you're not using your mind to its full capacity, as in retirement or underemployment. Intellectual stressors may leave us feeling mentally or emotionally overwhelmed and unable to problem-solve effectively.

Social stressors. Social stressors occur when one feels unduly pressured by certain groups such as family, coworkers, or friends to conform to their standards, beliefs, or behaviors. Anger and resentment are common reactions to social stressors.

Spiritual stressors. Any serious challenge to one's long-held personal, religious, or moral beliefs is a spiritual stressor. Anger, anxiety, and confusion are common responses.

When I started Active Wellness, I was not living a healthy life. I was under chronic stress at work and sleep deprived; as a wife and mother of three, I wanted more time to be with my family. I couldn't imagine how I was going to find time for myself. But, I knew I needed to do something, so I started Active Wellness.

Doing the Active Wellness Program helped me realize that in order to get healthier, I needed to reassess the priorities in my life. My pattern was indulging in food on the weekends as a "mini-vacation" away from the stress of the week. Over time I had gained weight, my energy dropped, I wasn't sleeping well, and I began getting terrible headaches.

Because of my limited time schedule, I worked on one small goal at a time. My first goal was to change to healthier foods for myself and my family. Soon after I started eating well and drinking plenty of water each day, my headaches disappeared. I realized then that the headaches were a result of not drinking enough water; I had been dehydrated.

Once I had my eating plan under way, I began to incorporate an exercise routine into my life. In order to exercise and incorporate time with my family, I instituted family walks, which became a regular routine; then I added a routine on a Stepper with weight training. While the exercise helped with my stress level, I knew I needed to institute a regular stress routine into my life because it was important for me to totally download and take the stress out of my mind and body, so I began to do deep breathing, meditate, and go to a yoga class. Finally, I decided that to truly bring balance to my life I needed to reassess my work life. I am now in a new position within the same company that aligns me with both my work and family priorities.

A year later, I feel on track with my life. I have more energy, I have dropped twenty-five pounds, I am more fit and strong. At times I feel like I exude energy. I am a healthier, happier person. I plan to do a four-mile run with my daughter in a few months, something I have never done in my life! Taking care of myself is now at the top of my priority list. Looking back, I am convinced that if I had not changed my life, I was headed down a path with some serious health risks. Active Wellness will pay off in so many ways. I highly recommend it.

◎ *Ann, age forty-two, weight loss 25 pounds, increased muscle mass, decreased stress*

The way we perceive things makes a difference in how our bodies respond to them. If you are going to a meeting or family gathering and not looking forward to it, this is your perspective in the moment. How you choose to view situations is really up to you. When you feel yourself getting stressed about a situation, try on a new perspective that also holds true for you and works with your belief system. Soon you will see that there are several different ways to approach the same circumstance and change your mindset and stress level.

By examining your own personal stressors, you can begin to observe how you respond to stress and then make conscious choices about changing your stress-coping methods.

Understanding Stress and How We Deal with It

How we respond to stress and how it affects our health depend on three factors: its intensity, its timing, and its duration.

Intensity of the Stress

Stress can be mild or severe. Assigning these labels to certain stress responses is difficult because the intensity of stress depends on your ability to adapt when confronted with a situation. The death of a loved one can clearly cause severe stress, but a person with strong coping abilities handles even a devastatingly stressful situation better than an individual with no coping skills. A seemingly mild stressful situation, such as losing one's car keys, may be a minor nuisance for one person, while throwing someone else into an emotional tailspin that ruins his or her day.

Timing of the Stress

You may find it more difficult to cope if a stress occurs after you have suffered a long line of previous stresses. Also, if stress occurs when you are dealing with an illness, it can have more serious repercussions than if you are healthy.

Duration of the Stress

Stress may also be acute (short term) or chronic (long term). A sudden and extremely threatening event or stimulus that appears for a short time is considered acute stress. A loud explosion close by, a near miss on the highway, a sudden blackout, or a suspicious crash downstairs while you are sleeping are examples of potentially acute stress.

Whether mild or severe, any stress that continues over a long period of time is considered chronic. Taking care of someone who is ill is an example of chronic stress; always worrying about money and coping with a high-pressure job are "milder" forms of chronic stress.

If you feel like every day is its own crisis, you may be suffering from chronic stress, which could be greatly harming your body. The charts below and on page 182 illustrate both the signs of chronic stress and the long-term effects that can occur when chronic stress isn't managed properly.

The "Fight or Flight" Response

Threatened with a stressor or chronic stress, the brain triggers the release of hormones that gear the body up to defend itself—either by fighting ("fight") or by running away ("flight"). These hormones spur body cells to release stored carbohydrates, fats, and proteins for energy to fuel the body. The circulatory system floods with adrenaline and nutrients. Metabolism increases, and all energy is switched to the muscles and brain. Muscular strength, physical endurance, mental clarity, and reaction times are greatly enhanced to ensure the survival of the body.

The list of physical responses goes on. Heart rate and blood pressure increase, so that the blood can transport nutrients and adrenaline as quickly as possible. Breathing also increases to help transport oxygen to the muscles at a greater rate. Body temperature rises to promote sweating. Digestion, sex drive, bone and tissue growth, and the immune system are suppressed to further conserve unneeded energy and channel "survival" energy to the mus-

Signs of Chronic Stress

- Irritability; fatigue
- Pounding heart
- Inability to concentrate
- Sweating
- Migraines; frequent headaches
- Nervous laughter
- Clumsiness; increased accidents
- Neck or lower back pain
- Clenched jaw; grinding teeth
- Increased use of alcohol and drugs to relax
- Difficulty sleeping; insomnia; bad dreams
- Nervous twitches
- Short fuse
- Feelings of anxiety, tension, moodiness
- Shallow breathing; shortness of breath
- Rapid speech

cles and brain. Memory cells are damaged in the brain, and fat is deposited at the waist instead of the hips and buttocks. Fat at the waist is a risk factor for heart disease, cancer, and other diseases.

These adaptations create a superb survival device of the human organism. Under normal circumstances, we are well equipped to handle a threatening situation. After a short-term acute crisis has been dealt with, the body quickly returns to normal functioning. When stress becomes chronic, however, and the body doesn't get a chance to return to normal, serious damage can occur.

Studies supported by the National Institutes of Health (NIH) suggest that chronic stress has significant effects on physical and emotional health. With chronic stress, the body remains in a modified but continual state of "fight or flight" readiness. Brain chemistry and the circulatory and immune systems never quite return to their normal functioning. Over time, this organic imbalance may cause chronic anxiety, depression, moodiness, and serious illness, including heart disease.

Managing Stress and Restoring Your Body's Balance

We all have stress in our lives at different times and to varying degrees. Our bodies and bodily systems are often in modified "stress response" or "fight or flight" states, fluctuating between healthy balance and stress-induced imbalance.

By learning a few improved ways to manage stress, you can help your body return to a healthy balance faster. And you'll find that the more you practice stress-management techniques, the more peaceful you will feel and the more mentally focused you will become. You can perform your day-to-day activities with greater ease, a clearer mind, and an increased sense of happiness. Paradoxically, by learning to manage stress and induce relaxation, you actually create healthier energy in your life.

The Relaxation Response

When you restore balance to your body and bring it to a relaxed state, you are inducing the relaxation response. This now-famous term, coined by Dr. Herbert Benson, was based on his studies at Harvard Medical School and is detailed in his book *The Relaxation Response*.

When your body is in a relaxed state, your blood pressure and heart rate are lower, your metabolism and muscle tension decrease, your body temperature drops, your body uses less oxygen and produces less carbon dioxide, and your hormones return to a balanced level.

When we are in deep relaxation, even our brain waves change in frequency. During the waking state, our brain emits beta waves. As we relax, beta waves change to slower alpha waves. During deep relaxation, alpha waves change to even slower theta waves (which are the brain waves during orgasm), but while you may feel deeply relaxed, mentally you are far more aware and alert.

The more you practice reaching this deep relaxation state, the easier time you have getting there. If you practice deep relaxation regularly, a general state of calmness and mental focus eventually infuses your everyday life.

ENGAGING IN "RELAXING" ACTIVITIES ISN'T ENOUGH

In order to achieve the benefits of a relaxed state, you must be aware of activities that actually enhance this state of being. Many times my clients tell me that they relax by reading a book, going to the movies, taking walks, or socializing with friends. While these kinds of activities are more relaxing than day-to-day chores and work, they do not help you experience deep relaxation.

THE BENEFITS OF MANAGING STRESS

- Increased energy
- Looking and feeling younger
- Increased power of concentration
- Increased feeling of happiness
- Increased awareness
- Improved sleep
- Enhanced performance
- Ease and efficiency in daily activities
- Improved sense of self-acceptance
- Improved flexibility

In order to achieve the relaxation response, you need a clear mind and relaxed muscles. According to this definition, exercise alone does not help induce relaxation. Exercise can reduce stress, but it doesn't help us relax. Why? Because our bodies and minds are not at rest while exercising. In order to achieve deep relaxation, you need to use a specific relaxation technique aimed at calming your body, mind, and spirit.

TECHNIQUES TO RELAX BODY AND SOUL

Just as there are different degrees of stress, there are different methods for managing stress and bringing your body into a balanced, relaxed state. Some techniques can be used easily—anytime, anywhere—to counteract a specific stressor. Others require a commitment of regular relaxation practice. For the rest of this chapter, the focus will be on four powerful techniques for managing stress and inducing deep relaxation: breathing exercises, meditation, visualization, and yoga and deep relaxation.

As you read about each technique and review the accompanying exercises, try to choose a stress-management method that particularly appeals to you. We include two types of methods here: those that can be done quickly, for on-the-spot stress relief; and those that require a commitment of thirty to sixty minutes but provide deeper and more lasting relaxation benefits.

Choose a practice that you are comfortable with, and one that is especially suited for your current level of stress. For example, if muscle tension is a major problem for you, yoga practice may be your best choice. If anxiety plagues you, breathing exercises and meditation may be better choices. Or you may wish to combine several practices, doing them at different times during the week. Your goal is to incorporate whatever stress-management methods you choose into your regular Active Wellness routine.

Breathing Exercises
BREATHING TO MANAGE STRESS AND RELAX

Have you ever stopped to think about how you breathe? Most of the time we don't have to think about breathing; it's an unconscious act that our bodies perform automatically. The quality of our breath reflects our emotions and state of mind. Many of us have breathing patterns that include gasping in fear or anxiously holding our breath. When we are stressed, we tend to take shallow, rapid breaths.

Examining how you breathe under different circumstances can help you determine when you are stressed, angry, happy, enraged, tense. Is your breathing rapid and shallow or deep and slow? Rapid and shallow breaths are associated with feelings of fatigue and stress. Count how many breaths you take in one minute. If your count falls between sixteen and twenty, you probably are breathing rapidly and from your chest and are underutilizing your lung capacity. This type of breathing inhibits the uptake of oxygen. The extreme example of this is hyperventilating, which can actually trigger the stress response.

We can learn to regulate our breathing to induce relaxation by breathing diaphragmatically. Diaphragmatic breathing, which originates in the belly, is an easy technique to learn and one that you can use anytime. Diaphragmatic breathing was the way we naturally breathed as infants. The emphasis is on the exhaled breath rather than the inhaled breath. As you inhale, your diaphragm moves downward, expanding your lungs. As you exhale, the diaphragm contracts, compressing the lungs and forcing the old air out. This movement gives you full use of your lungs, both to take in oxygen and to release carbon dioxide.

Diaphragmatic breathing is an excellent de-stressing tool and a great way to relax, whether you use it by itself as a means to calm down after a hectic day or as part of a longer yoga and meditation routine. Generally, with diaphragmatic breathing you take fewer and deeper breaths, averaging about six to eight breaths per minute—but don't hold yourself to this. Do what feels comfortable. This type of breathing isn't difficult to learn, but it takes focused energy and awareness when you're beginning. With regular practice, it becomes the norm.

LEARNING TO BREATHE FROM YOUR DIAPHRAGM

This simple exercise helps you learn the process of diaphragmatic breathing. Once you feel comfortable with this process, you can start to incorporate it into your regular breathing process.

Step 1: Become aware of your breathing. Sit or lie down in a quiet room with your hand placed on your abdomen.

Step 2: Breathe normally. Inhale and exhale through your nose. Notice if your abdomen fills with air as you inhale. On the inhalation, your belly should expand slightly on its own. Try to relax your abdominal muscles; you'll get the most effective breath from a relaxed abdomen.

Step 3: The hand that is resting on your abdomen should rise up with your belly as you inhale and go down as you exhale. Focus on creating this effect, feeling your abdomen expand and your hand rise as you inhale and then feeling your abdomen contract and your hand drop as you exhale.

If you initially find it difficult to practice diaphragmatic breathing, give yourself time. Remember that this was how you were born breathing; eventually it will come back to you. Some clients take several weeks to learn diaphragmatic breathing. Once they do, however, it becomes their favorite of the relaxation techniques, as it is easy to do and can be done anywhere.

MINDFULNESS BREATHING AS RELAXATION PRACTICE

Mindfulness breathing involves consciously focusing on your breath for a specific amount of time. You can do this for short periods of time, at various moments throughout the day, to relax yourself. Or, preferably, set aside a designated time and place to regularly practice mindfulness breathing as part of your stress-management program. Mindfulness breathing also offers a great way to start learning the practice of meditation: Focusing on the breath, and the breath alone, is a common meditative technique.

FIVE-MINUTE MINDFULNESS BREATHING EXERCISE This mindfulness breathing exercise is a wonderful way to begin or end your day. Try to find a safe, comfortable place for this exercise, so you can really relax.

Step 1: Set aside at least five minutes for this breathing practice.

Step 2: Get yourself into a comfortable position, either sitting or lying down, with your arms by your sides. (Lying down is more restful to the body.)

Step 3: Close your eyes.

Step 4: Begin breathing, focusing your attention on your breath as you inhale and exhale. Keep bringing your attention back to your breath when it wanders.

Step 5: As you breathe, take long, deep inhalations and exhalations, preferably through your nose. In the beginning, you may find it helpful to count to 3 during the inhaled breath and count to 4 during the exhaled breath. By doing this, you exhale more slowly, which helps you cleanse your lungs and further relax.

Step 6: When you are ready to finish your breathing session, slowly resume normal breathing and open your eyes.

Meditation

Meditation is a way to nourish your soul and calm your mind. It is a way of taking time to focus in a quiet, peaceful, and accepting manner. The practice of meditation helps to induce relaxation, enhance concentration, increase mental alertness, and promote creativity.

There are many different ways to meditate. Because each person has a different learning style, I've included a variety of meditation methods. For example, some people respond to visual images, while others relate better to sound. You may want to experiment before deciding which works best for you. Although you can achieve effective meditation using a variety of techniques, the most important factor for choosing a particular type of meditation is your own comfort level with the technique.

FOCUSED MEDITATION

An excellent practice for inducing deep relaxation and increasing mental clarity and awareness is focused meditation. With this type of meditation, you focus on one thing, whether it's your breath, a word, a phrase, an object, an image, or a sound. When you first begin practicing focused meditation, you may have difficulty staying focused on just one thing. You may feel easily distracted, as if your mind is going off in twenty different directions. With practice, however, you can learn how to remain so focused within your meditation that time seems to stand still. This happened to me when I first "got into" a meditative state. I sat down to meditate for ten to fifteen minutes and before I knew it, I had meditated for more than half an hour.

Before you begin your meditation, plan to follow these few simple guidelines:

* Wear comfortable, loose clothing or loosen your waistband and shirt cuffs.
* Choose a calm and quiet place to meditate where you won't be disturbed. If necessary, take the phone off the hook.
* Establish a regular time and place for meditating every day. Many people choose to practice first thing in the morning or right before going to bed. I personally recommend meditating first thing in the morning, which helps you start your day with a clear, calm, and focused mind.

BEGINNING YOUR MEDITATION Sit or kneel with your spine straight. For sitting positions, you may use the floor or a chair.

For floor position: Sit cross-legged on the floor with your spine straight, a hand on each knee, and palms facing upward.

For chair position: Sit upright in a chair with your feet flat on the floor, spine straight, a hand on each knee, and palms facing upward.

For kneeling position: Kneel on the floor with your spine straight, a hand resting on each knee, and palms facing upward.

Hand and finger positioning: With palms facing upward, gently touch your thumb to your index finger. By uniting your thumb and index finger, you, in effect, "close a circuit" and keep the flow of energy circulating throughout your body.

BREATH-FOCUSED MEDITATION Close your eyes and begin deep breathing through your nose, focusing on your breath as it travels in and out of your body. If it helps you maintain your focus, count to 3 as you inhale and then to 4 as you exhale. At first, you may find yourself easily distracted by outside noises and your own thoughts, random images, and feelings. Observe any thoughts, images, feelings, and distractions that come up during meditation, but try not to become "attached" to them. Picture them as clouds floating through your mind. Observe them calmly, but let them go and return to focusing on your breath. As you continue your meditation practice, you will find it easier to remain focused on your breath.

If you are a beginner to meditation, start out by meditating for five minutes at a time. Gradually increase your meditation time each week. By beginning slowly, you give your body a chance to become comfortable with the meditation posture and discipline. If your body is uncomfortable, you may have difficulty remaining still and focusing your mind. You may choose to continue doing breath-focused meditation exclusively, or you may want to try another type of focused meditation.

WORD-FOCUSED MEDITATION In this type of meditation, a continually repeated word or phrase (also called a "mantra") becomes the focus of your meditation. You may repeat the word or phrase silently to yourself, timing it with the inhalation and exhalation of your breath, or you may say the word or phrase aloud, but quietly. What is important is to select a word or phrase that has a strong personal meaning for you and is also uplifting and positive. Words such as *love, light, hope,* and *relax* are excellent choices for word-focused meditation. A phrase such as "I wish all living creatures love and kindness" is also a good choice.

IMAGE-FOCUSED MEDITATION An object or image offers a visual focus that may help sharpen and increase your awareness. You should choose a simple object or image—a beautiful stone, a crystal, a candle, a plant, or a small painting. Place the object or image about one to two feet away from you. Begin deep breathing, but do not close your eyes. Instead, focus on the object or image in front of you for a few minutes, until you feel calm and centered. Then close your eyes, if you wish, and become aware of any thoughts or images that enter your mind.

SOUND-FOCUSED MEDITATION Choose an outside sound—the singing of birds, the rustling of leaves, the laughter of children—and use this sound as your focus when you begin deep breathing. Try to focus on the unique timbre and various facets of the sound. You may also choose to use a passage of music as your focus, concentrating on hearing each sound as a separate note. You can use meditation tapes, recorded natural sounds, or chanting as sounds for your meditation. Do not become attached to the sound; simply allow it to pass in and out of your meditative space.

MINDFULNESS MEDITATION

This type of meditation focuses on being aware of each moment. It involves observing the things that we do or that occur in our lives moment by moment. Mindfulness meditation is a process of fine-tuning your awareness of the present and learning how to become absorbed in each moment of your life as it occurs. You can practice mindfulness meditation anywhere and anytime, such as sitting in your office, eating dinner, or walking in the park. As you focus your attention and awareness on each facet of the particular moment you are experiencing, you will begin to notice and observe things that you were not aware of before. This is a particularly illuminating exercise when done while eating.

While meditation is frequently incorporated into yoga and breathing exercises, it can also stand on its own as a means of training your mind to relax and focus. If you do not have time to meditate at home, try taking time for meditation in your office. Shut your office door and hold all calls for the time you have allotted to your meditation. It may be difficult to meditate in your desk chair. Since this is where you do your work, it's not a spot associated with relaxation. Instead, choose another comfortable spot in your office where you can sit calmly to begin meditation.

VISUALIZATION

Visualization is a technique whereby you picture a specific image in your mind as a way to change your thoughts. It can alter your subconscious, help you relax, and even promote healing. Visualizing an image in your mind has a very powerful influence on your emotions, one that is far more potent than just reading or hearing about the image. It has been proven that various types of imagery affect breathing, heart rate, blood pressure, sexual arousal, hormone levels in the blood, and the immune system.

Take a moment now to compare how differently your feelings are affected by the idea described in the statement below and, after that, the impression evoked in your mind by the image that follows.

Statement: It is a beautiful day.
Now, close your eyes, take three deep breaths, and visualize the following image.

Image: The sun is shining. The sky is blue. The air feels crisp and fresh. Birds are flying overhead.

You probably noticed that the image was much stronger than the statement, or perhaps reading the statement caused you to instantly picture an image.

Testimonial

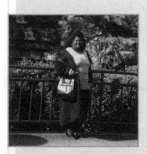

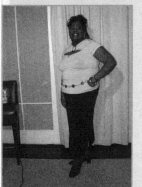

I never realized how much stress played a role in my eating until I began Active Wellness. Every time I would feel stressed, either from work, a bad relationship, or my graduate studies, I would overeat. By using stress-management techniques I learned from Active Wellness, I now have an awareness of recognizing when I am feeling stressed and the tools to stop it from sabatoging my healthy lifestyle program. Depending on where I am—at work or at home—I either use breathing, journaling, aromatherapy, or yoga to help me release the energy from my frustration, stress, and disappointments. I feel more balanced now, which stops me from using food like chips and sweets to soothe my nerves. Having greater self-awareness helps me feel in control of my actions—this is a very powerful feeling. I am on my way to losing more weight, having lost the first twenty-five pounds. I know I can do it, because not only have I taken control of how stress affects me and learned how to discharge it, but I am also exercising regularly and tracking my eating. I am more confident, I feel more attractive, and I definitely have a higher self-esteem. This has been a great program for me. I now have a new mantra—nothing is going to get in the way of "the Active Wellness me."

Lisa, age thirty, weight loss 25 pounds, decreased stress, increased self-confidence

The image affects how we feel; the words are a tool by which our body and our mind communicate. You are probably more familiar with the practice of visualization than you realize. For example, before trying anything new, we usually try to see ourselves doing it first. This is visualization and it is powerful, particularly when done in combination with meditation. In fact, images sent to your subconscious while you are in a meditative state are twenty times more effective than visualizations done in the conscious state.

This ability is linked to the fact that there are two sides to our brain, the left and the right, which function together. The right brain is responsible for responding to images, and the left brain is the logical side of the brain. By using visualization in meditation, you can use the images that naturally come to you to tap into the right brain's "knowledge" of the big picture of an event or feeling. This helps you discover feelings that would not have been unearthed by logical thinking alone. Discovering these hidden needs and desires, about which you may not have been aware, can be very valuable.

In fact, because visualization helps me uncover my "gut feelings" about specific situations, it is one of my own favorite ways to meditate. When you follow your instincts, you are more connected to your inner voice and more likely to make a balanced decision between your logical side and your emotional, instinctive side. I find this very valuable in both my business and my personal life. You can also purchase guided meditations, which lead you through the visualization process and show you how to incorporate the practice of visualization within your meditation practice.

Yoga and Deep Relaxation

The practice of yoga unites the techniques of breathing and relaxation through a series of gentle stretching exercises called "poses" or "postures." In fact, the Sanskrit word *yoga* means "union" or "yoking." Yoga itself is an ancient practice designed to link body, mind, and spirit in a balanced and relaxed state of well-being.

To have a free and relaxed mind, you need a flexible and relaxed body. The various yoga poses do just this by relieving muscle tension and promoting physical and mental well-being. I like to think of yoga as self-massage. It is even better than having a massage partner, since once you learn the poses you can practice them anywhere by yourself. Although practicing yoga is not considered a strenuous workout, I recommend that you check with your physician before you start practicing it (as you should with any new type of physical activity). A basic yoga practice, consisting of a series of poses that targets all the major muscle groups, is explained and illustrated on the following pages. However, I highly recommend that you take a yoga class or work with a private instructor when you first start out. An instructor can teach you proper breathing techniques for each pose and can show you how to make a smooth transition from one pose to the next. When practicing your yoga poses, please remember that you should not force your body into any position. Instead, try to feel a comfortable stretch. The goal in yoga is to improve flexibility, not to increase tension by exceeding your body's limits. Use your breathing to help release your muscles by inhaling and exhaling as you flex.

The order in which the yoga poses are explained is deliberate, so practice each pose in successive order. The overall organization of the poses is intended to help balance the left and right sides of your body. Set aside a specific time for your practice—sixty to ninety minutes is ideal—in a quiet and relaxed environment where you will not be interrupted, although fifteen to twenty minutes is better than not practicing at all. Also, practicing yoga on an empty stomach is best.

BEGINNING YOUR YOGA PRACTICE

Begin your practice standing tall, with your feet together and your arms by your sides.

1. The Corpse: This is a relaxation pose. Lie down on your back with your feet about eighteen inches apart and turned outward slightly. Place your arms at your sides, about six inches from your hips, with palms facing up. Close your eyes and breathe deeply, slowly inhaling and exhaling. Remain in this pose for at least 1 minute. While you are in this pose, use your breath to release any tension or tightness by focusing your mind on the area of discomfort and releasing it when you exhale. Hold this pose for 1 minute.

2. The Cat: To begin the Cat pose, slowly roll over onto your stomach with a gentle movement. Begin this pose on your hands and knees. Breathe in slowly and deeply while you hollow your back and look up. You should feel a gentle stretch, but no strain. Exhale and tuck in your head to your chest, rounding your back so your spine curves up, arching your back in the opposite direction. Repeat this pose 3 to 5 times, coordinating your breath with the up-and-down stretching of your spine.

3. The Child: Kneel with your legs together and sit back on your heels; bend from your hips and extend your upper body over your knees. Place your forehead down and your arms to your sides, palms upward. Rest in this pose for 30 to 60 seconds, then slowly sit up.

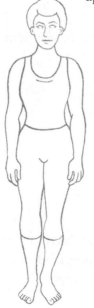

4. The Mountain: Stand with your arms by your sides, palms facing inward and feet together; balance yourself equally on both feet. Keep your spine straight and imagine your head being lifted straight up. As you stand, inhale and exhale slowly and deeply. Hold this pose for 60 seconds, or less if uncomfortable.

5. The Rag Doll: From a standing position, gradually bend over, hanging your head down. Cradle one arm in the other by holding each arm with the opposite hand. Hold this pose for 30 seconds, then slowly stand up, raising your head last. Repeat this pose 1 time. Return to a standing position.

6. The Tree (This is a more advanced pose—if you choose to skip this pose, proceed to pose 7, the Cobra.): Stand tall and straight. Lift and bend one leg so the foot of the bent leg is resting on the opposite thigh. Reach your arms upward and over your head. Interlace your fingers, keeping your index fingers free and pointing upward. Hold for 30 to 60 seconds. Repeat with the other leg.

7. The Cobra: Lie on your stomach with your hands by your sides. Bending your elbows, place your hands flat on the floor next to your shoulders. Slowly touch your forehead to the floor. Make sure your elbows are pointed toward your feet. Inhale as you push down with your hands and look up. Continue to inhale as you raise your head and chest, trying to lift only your upper body (see diagram). When you reach as far as you comfortably can go with your abdomen and chest, take a deep breath, and exhale as you slowly return to the floor. Repeat this pose 3 times. When finished, rest on the floor with your head turned and your arms comfortably by your sides.

8. The Half Locust: Lie on the floor on your stomach. In preparation for the Half Locust, place your arms under your thighs. Lift one leg up, pressing down with your arms for support and squeezing your buttocks. Raise the lifted leg outward and upward, lifting through your heel and toes. Press down both hips equally. Return your leg slowly to the floor. Repeat with the other leg. Repeat this sequence 2 times for both legs. Hold your leg up for 30 seconds.

9. The Full Locust: At the end of the Half Locust, raise both legs together for a Full Locust. This sequence may be repeated two times. Hold your legs up for 30 seconds.

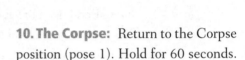

10. The Corpse: Return to the Corpse position (pose 1). Hold for 60 seconds.

11. The Knee Down Twist: Lie on your back with your arms extended out. Inhale and place your right foot on your left knee. Exhale, turn your head to the right, and bring your right knee toward the floor (see diagram). Release slowly, then repeat on the other side.

12. The Full Forward Bend: Sit with both legs directly in front of you, feet together and back straight. Inhaling, slowly bring both arms straight over your head. Exhale as you bend from your hips and grab your ankles. Drop your head and neck. Hold this pose for 30 to 60 seconds. Inhale as you raise your torso to return to a seated position. Repeat this pose 2 times.

13. The Corpse: Return to the Corpse position (pose 1). Hold for 60 seconds.

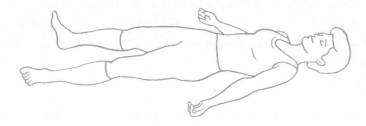

14. The Shoulder Stand (This is a more advanced pose—if you choose to skip this pose, proceed to pose 15, the Bridge.): Lie on your back with your arms along your sides. Make sure that your feet are together. Inhale and slowly lift both legs until they are at a right angle to your back. Place both of your hands on your lower back to support your body. Inhale and extend your legs straight up (see diagram). Make sure to keep your chin tucked into your chest. Hold the pose for 30 seconds, or as long as you are comfortable, and then slowly return to the relaxation pose. Take several deep breaths.

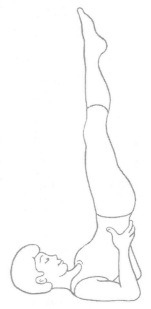

15. The Bridge: Lie on your back, knees bent, palms on the floor. Inhale as you slowly raise your pelvis and squeeze your buttocks. Press your arms and shoulders to the floor. Exhale as you lower your pelvis back down to the floor. Hold this pose for 30 seconds, breathing slowly and evenly. Repeat this pose 2 times.

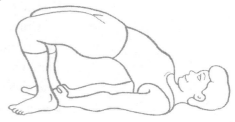

16. The Corpse: This pose is for Body Scan and Deep Relaxation. Return to the Corpse position (pose 1).

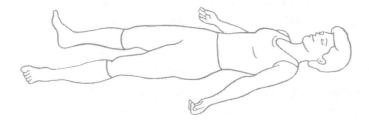

Body Scan: Remain in the Corpse pose and continue breathing for 5 minutes. Take a minute to mentally scan your body from your toes to your head, checking for any tension. Wherever you feel tension, picture that area of your body. As you exhale, imagine the tension disappearing from that part of your body.

Deep Relaxation: Raise your legs two inches from the floor and tense them. Then release them and let them fall to the floor. Let your feet lie still as though they were too heavy to lift. Raise your right arm and clench your fist. Then spread your fingers out and release your hand and arm, letting them fall to the floor. Repeat the same movements with your left arm and fist. Then allow your hands and arms to lie still and "be absorbed by the floor," as though they were too heavy to lift.

Raise your buttocks from the floor and tense your muscles. Then relax, allowing your buttocks to drop to the floor. Take a deep breath. Inhale and fill your stomach with as much air as possible, then let out the air with a sigh. Raise your back and chest from the floor and tense them. Then relax your muscles and let yourself fall back to the floor. Pull your shoulders up to your ears and tense your neck. Then release them and let your shoulders fall back to their original position.

Crunch and tense your facial muscles, open your eyes wide, stick out your tongue, and stretch your face. Then let go and relax. Roll your neck from side to side to find a comfortable place for your head. Then allow your body to lie still. Picture a warm wave of relaxation entering at your toes and traveling up your body through your legs to your back, stomach, arms, neck, face, and jaw, finally quieting your mind in a peaceful state of calm relaxation. You may lie in this position for several minutes.

To waken your body, gently begin to move your arms and legs. Then slowly come to a sitting position. You may, at this stage, want to practice a short meditation before you resume your daily activities.

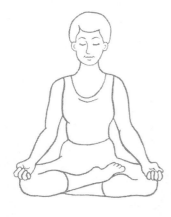

17. The Lotus: To finish your stress-management routine, you can return to the Lotus pose (meditation pose) and close with a short meditation. To sit in the Lotus pose, cross your legs; bring one leg close to your body and the other leg to the opposite thigh. It's best if your knees don't touch the floor. Sit with your spine straight and your arms resting on your knees, palms faced upward. Close your eyes, inhale, then exhale slowly and begin your meditation.

Stress-Management Routines for the Office, Train, or Plane

Many stress-management routines can be adapted to use at work or when traveling on a train or plane. You'll find stress management particularly beneficial when you are on a business trip, because it helps diminish the stress associated with airline traveling, meeting deadlines, irregular hours, and living out of a suitcase. Below are some simple breathing, stretching, and yoga exercises, all of which can be done while you are seated. You can do each of the exercise sets at different times during the day. You may prefer to combine all three components of the routine into one mini stress-management workout, which is especially beneficial when you travel.

BREATHING EXERCISE

Take three deep meditating breaths to relax. Repeat 2 or 3 times. You can also use a stress-management audiocassette tape to practice deep breathing or listen to relaxing meditation music.

STRETCHING EXERCISE

Stretch your neck by gently rotating your head from the front to the right side, to the back, and to the left side in a circular motion. First, look straight ahead, then drop your chin to your chest and allow your neck to stretch for approximately 15 seconds. Slowly move your head to the right so that your ear is touching or is horizontal to your right shoulder. Remember to stretch only to a point that is comfortable for you. Now slowly rotate your head toward the back and then continue around to your left shoulder. Repeat this stretch 3 times.

GENTLE YOGA EXERCISES

Sitting yoga postures energize you and relieve some of the tension caused by work or by sitting for long periods of time. Follow the diagrams shown for each posture.

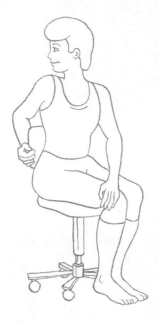

Seated spine twist: Sitting straight in a chair with a back, with your feet flat on the floor, place your left hand on the outside of your right knee and your right hand on the back of your seat. Look forward and gently inhale as you turn toward the right, twisting your spine as far as possible without strain and exhaling as you twist. Repeat this 3 times. Perform the exercise twisting to the left, switching hands so that your left hand is on the back of your seat.

Seated knee squeeze: Sit straight up and forward in your seat. Breathe in and lift your right knee up toward your chest. Exhale, inhale, grab your knee with both hands, and hold your breath while gently squeezing your knee toward your chest. Exhale as you release your leg and return it with one smooth movement back to the floor. (If you have joint problems with your knees, grab your inside thigh instead to reduce the pressure placed on your knee.) Repeat the exercise 3 times. Then switch legs to perform the exercise 4 times.

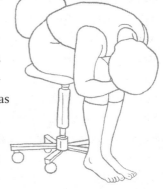

Overhead stretch for shoulders, arms, and upper back: Hold your right arm up and bend it behind your head, grasping your elbow with your left hand and gently pulling the elbow downward until you feel an easy tension in the shoulder or back of the upper arm. Breathe and hold the stretch for 30 seconds. Do not force this stretch. Repeat the exercise 3 times with each arm.

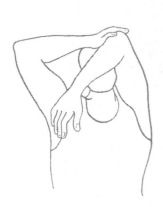

Lower-back stretch: To end your stretches you can do a lower-back stretch by sitting forward in your chair and leaning over your knees, as shown in the diagram. This releases the tension in your back. Make sure you hang your neck down to release the tension there as well. Look toward your feet. Hold this stretch for 45 seconds. Breathe throughout the stretch. When you are ready to return to a seated position, you can use the seat of your chair or your thighs for support as you push up.

End your routine by taking three deep breaths, inhaling and exhaling through your nose.

Travel never needs to be tedious again if you think of it as a special time to devote to yourself and your health.

Creating Stress-Free Living and Working Environments

Feng Shui

If you have ever been in a room that felt stuffy and tight, you probably felt uncomfortable and even drained of energy. On the other hand, in a spacious, light-filled, airy room with a good view, you probably felt energized and happy. Creating energy in a living or working environment is the goal of Feng Shui (pronounced "fung shway"), the ancient Chinese art of the placement of buildings, rooms, objects, and color to promote positive energy, happiness, and prosperity. In fact, the Chinese ideogram for Feng Shui means "under the canopy of heaven." There are many excellent books available if you want to learn about Feng Shui in depth. Here, we are introducing some Feng Shui basics for creating stress-free home and work environments.

In Feng Shui, the type of energy created in an environment depends on the intended use. The energy in a home environment, for example, should be calming, while the energy in a retail store should be stimulating enough to promote business.

The first step in using Feng Shui to reenergize your home or office is to look at any areas of your environment that disturb you. Is there a lot of clutter in one area? Do you have a brick wall for a view? Does your home or office feel tight and closed off? Focus on the feeling you get when you walk into your home or office: Is it a good feeling or an uncomfortable one? Feng Shui is based on the Chinese philosophy of yin and yang, whereby two separate but complementary elemental energies of the universe are constantly interacting with each other. Together, they are the components of qi (pronounced "chee"), the fundamental life force that lives within everything. Yin is feminine energy and yang is masculine energy. Yin is cold, yang is hot. Yin is the earth, moon, darkness, and death. Yang is the heavens, sun, light, and life. One cannot exist without the other. Both are necessary for harmonious balance.

Balance and order, based on the yin-yang dynamic, are the fundamental tenets of Feng Shui and of creating stress-free environments. Rooms are designed and objects are placed in them based on the goal of balancing yin and yang qualities. In Feng Shui, design and placement are also dependent on geographical direction. For example, a southerly direction is associated with fortune, the color red, and summer; a northerly direction is linked to business, death, the color black, and winter; the westerly direction is associated with children, purity, the color white, and autumn; and the easterly direction symbolizes family, health, the color green, and spring.

SUGGESTIONS FOR HOME AND OFFICE

As you walk into your home, what is the first thing that greets you? Is it cheerful or depressing? Hopefully you enter a well-lighted and open environment. However, if you walk into a room and find yourself facing a wall, you may feel stifled and uncomfortable. Placing a mirror or a painting of a landscape on that wall opens up the environment. Adding warm light to a dark foyer brings good energy into that environment, as does placing lights, mirrors, and pictures in a narrow hallway. As you go through your home, room by room, look for areas with clutter, darkness, narrowness, or poor views.

How you decorate a room also sets a mood. If a room is cold and uninviting, visitors will feel uncomfortable. When you are decorating or rearranging furniture in a home or office, keep in mind that it is important to leave space between furniture and to eliminate clutter. It helps to visualize the flow of positive energy beginning at the doorway of the room. That energy then flows toward groupings of furniture, slowly meanders through the room, and then leaves via another door or window. Because positive energy enters at the door, avoid obstructing the doorway with any furniture.

For an office environment, the ideal location for your desk is facing the door, positioned far enough inside the office so that you can see the entire room from your desk. Plants and flowers contribute to the positive energy in an environment, as does a good view. Any furniture that has edges is thought to cut into positive energy in a negative way. Try to avoid having any corners from bookcases or furniture face you directly. Good lighting is important, but glaring lights should be avoided. Clear thinking is obscured with clutter, so avoid clutter or try to organize it.

If the energy in a room is active, such as in a living room, it is more yang than yin. To balance the yang energy in an active room, try using yin touches throughout the room, such as throw pillows and cooling elements such as plants. Combining dark and light colors will also help achieve more harmonious energy and greater balance in the room.

COLOR The colors you use throughout your home can greatly affect your well-being. Color can influence appetite, the autonomic nervous system, muscular tension, and emotional reactions. Surround yourself with colors that suit your emotions. In general, many of our emotional associations with color come from the natural world around us. For example, red is associated with fire, green with trees, and blue with the sky.

Also, remember that you are striving for a harmonious balance with color, based on the same yin-yang principle of energy used in Feng Shui. Yin colors are cooling, contrasting, and astringent. They include blues, indigo, and violet. Yang colors are warm, arousing, and vitalizing. They include red, orange, and yellow. If you want to learn more about the use of color to create a balanced and stress-free environment, you can find specific books devoted to Feng Shui and the use of colors for each room of your home.

LIGHTING In general, a well-lighted room feels more comfortable. However, choose carefully what types of lighting you use. A glaring overhead light that is hard on the eyes is not as welcoming and soothing as a lamp with a warm-glowing bulb. Fluorescent light is much harder to live with than soft light.

SCENT (A.K.A. AROMATHERAPY) Aromatherapy is the ancient art of using the healing power of aromatic essential oils to balance the mind and body. Essential oils are distilled from organic plant sources, including flowers and the leaves, bark, and gum of trees.

Smell is a potent influence on how we feel and act. Here is one example of just how potent smell can be. When I was trying to sell my home, a real-estate broker suggested that I make baked apples when clients were coming to view my home. She explained that the scent of baked apples invariably gives a cozy, warm feeling to a house.

The right scent can trigger your brain to stimulate your endocrine and hormonal systems in positive ways, which help you relax and de-stress. While more than 300 essential oils are available for home use, you should need no more than 10 to 15 different scents. Essential oils can be found in many stores and also come in scented-candle form. They offer a great way to quickly scent any room, even your bathroom. In the sidebar at left, you'll find a list of the most popular and effective essential oils.

Oils can be used during baths or showers, in inhalers or light-bulb diffusers, or as rubs or personal perfumes. But before you begin to experiment with oils, try a patch test on your skin to make sure you do not have an allergic reaction to any oils. Also, some oils should not be used if you are pregnant or photosensitive, so read the label on the bottle carefully or consult an aromatherapist.

Essential oils are also extremely volatile, so be sure to store them in a dark bottle in a cool and dark location. When essential oils are blended with a good base oil, they can keep for several months. There are many aromatherapy books available that can help you learn how to make a variety of skin-care and home-care products from essential oils.

SOUND Finally, don't forget the auditory senses. Sounds are directly linked to our nervous system and therefore can greatly affect our level of relaxation and stimulation.

Music therapy is an emerging field. Two excellent books on the subject are *Healing Imagery & Music* (CD included!) by Carol A. Bush and *The Sound of Healing* by Judith Pinkerton. Both books contain marvelous discussions about how various types of music affect us differently, both physically and emotionally. Loud and fast music is stimulating to our senses and increases the action of our autonomic nervous system. Slow and soft sounds are soothing and relaxing, decreasing the autonomic response and thereby helping decrease blood pressure, heart rate, and respiration.

When selecting music to help you relax, one of the most important criteria is your personal reaction to the piece of music. How much you like the music is the best indicator of how well the music will make you feel and how

Calming: Cedarwood, Chamomile, Frankincense, Geranium, Lavender, Lemongrass, Orange, Patchouli, Rosewood, Sandalwood, Ylang-Ylang

Uplifting: Basil, Bergamot, Ginger, Lavender, Lemon, Lime, Neroli, Peppermint, Rose, Rosemary

Clear Thinking: Black Pepper, Juniper, Lemon, Peppermint, Rosemary, Rosewood, Sage

Sensuality: Basil, Bergamot, Cedarwood, Frankincense, Geranium, Ginger, Jasmine, Juniper, Lavender, Lemongrass, Lime, Neroli, Orange, Patchouli, Rose, Sandalwood, Ylang-Ylang

much it will help you relax. Music is also an invaluable aid to meditation and visualization practice. Many musical audiocassettes and CDs are designed specifically for use during meditation and visualization.

THE BEDROOM AS A SPECIAL PLACE The main rule for positioning your bed is to avoid placing the foot of the bed in such a manner that your feet face the door. The Chinese refer to this as the "death position" because traditionally the dead were placed with their feet facing the door to allow them easier access to heaven. Since sleep is so highly regarded as a time of healing, several similar Feng Shui rules apply to the bedroom. For example, mirrors shouldn't face the bed, as they could scare your spirit at night. Also, furniture with sharp edges should never be placed so that the sharp edges are pointed at the sleeping person.

Avoid clutter in order to allow the maximum positive healing energy to circulate throughout the room. If you are using a portion of your bedroom for storing boxes, books, and extra clothing, these objects interrupt the flow of energy. Similarly, using the space under your bed for storage creates stagnant energy over your bed.

For those of you who can't avoid the placement of your bed and furniture in precarious positions, solutions to these problems are available. You can hang a crystal sphere or wind chime from the ceiling between the bed and the door to lessen the negative energy. Folding screens and plants also divert the flow of negative energy. And, if possible, try to create an enjoyable view to wake up to, such as a picture, plants, or a pleasant view through the window.

Another tenet of Feng Shui is using "conscious intent" to achieve your goals. Meditating right before sleep about your aspirations and goals is highly recommended. Write down your thoughts and dreams before you go to bed, which is considered a cleansing ritual in Feng Shui, and then focus on your goals right before falling asleep. By focusing on your goals and dreams just before sleeping, you are closing the day with positive energy—a great way to begin your night.

THE KITCHEN AND BATHROOM According to Feng Shui philosophy, a well-lighted kitchen enhances the flow of good energy. This concept is especially important because the kitchen is often a place where clutter easily accumulates. Try to eliminate clutter, or it may stagnate the good energy flow. That stagnant energy, in turn, affects the food you prepare and eat in the kitchen.

The bathroom is a tricky room to arrange according to Feng Shui principles. Water, which in Feng Shui is symbolic of business, wealth, and success, is also something that gets flushed out of the bathroom daily. Therefore, even more attention should be paid to the flow of positive energy in and around the room. Keep the room clean and uncluttered. The bathroom is a mostly yin environment, so adding yang touches—warm colors and candlelight—promotes balance and positive energy.

Finally, if the bathroom is facing the front door or situated near the kitchen or in the central part of your house, hang a mirror outside the bathroom door to deflect any negative energy from spilling over into these other environments.

You've nearly completed the Active Wellness Program, realized many of your short-term goals, and are well on the way to experiencing your long-term goal of lifelong wellness. It's time to take a breather and congratulate yourself for a job well done. To reward yourself, move on to Step 7, where you will learn some new techniques for nurturing yourself and maintaining your successes.

Main Points to Ways to Manage Stress

✔ Stress can interfere with the balance in our lives and impact our eating patterns, mood, sleep, and immunity. Learning to manage stress affects your mind, body, and spirit. It helps bring a centered, balanced feeling into your life from which all life activities can emanate.

✔ There are many types of stressors. Once you determine where your stress is coming from, it is easier to recognize it and control it.

✔ Using the techniques of breathing, meditation, and yoga you can integrate stress management and relaxation into your life wherever you are.

✔ You can do simple yoga stretches at home or in your office. Active Wellness gives you an easy routine to follow so you can begin learning the benefits of yoga, relaxing the mind and body.

✔ You can also manage the stress associated with your environment by using relaxation tools that address your senses and Feng Shui to address the space in a room.

7

Maintaining Active Wellness for a Lifetime

AS YOU'VE TAKEN each step in the Active Wellness journey, you've gained a new awareness of your health, your behaviors, and your thoughts. You have acquired powerful new tools to build an individualized program of optimal health and well-being. With your new awareness and new tools, you have begun making some profound changes in your life. An integral component to maintaining those changes is nurturing and rewarding yourself for your positive efforts. Have you been rewarding yourself for your successes, however small? If not, what are you waiting for?

Taking Inventory of Your Successes

Back at the beginning of your wellness journey, you set some short- and long-term health goals. Take a moment now to recall those goals. Take a personal inventory of how you've changed. Have you achieved some of your goals? Have you adopted any new behaviors? Have you conquered any old, unhealthy habits? How do you feel—body, mind, and soul?

Right now, write down some of the changes you've made and the successes you've enjoyed.

Goals I've reached and changes I've made:

_____

_____

_____

_____

_____

As you traveled along the Active Wellness path, you may have noticed what happened as you applied yourself more to a specific goal: It became easier to practice your new behavior in the short run—and to achieve that goal in a short amount of time.

Long-term changes (the ones that are meant to last a lifetime), however, require renewed vigilance, time, patience, and practice. As you progress and mature along the wellness path, you will continue to use your new awareness and health skills to replace unhealthy behaviors with healthy ones. But to truly feel in control of your health and stride purposefully forward toward a lifetime of wellness, you need some new tools as touchstones for your journey.

New Tools for a Lifetime of Active Wellness

COMMIT TO YOURSELF

The very act of taking responsibility for your own health actually furthers your good health. Research shows that people who care and nurture other people and things—loved ones, pets, plants—are healthier and happier than those who don't. Making a compassionate commitment to care for others gives us a sense of purpose and enhances our self-worth and well-being. Making a commitment to care for yourself will give you this same sense of purpose, which can enhance your health and self-esteem. How much more powerful is a compassionate commitment to our own good health?

USE POSITIVE REINFORCEMENT

Nurture yourself with rewards and self-care, which are powerful agents of positive reinforcement. Rewards can come in the form of a gift, personal treat, or special event. An example of self-care involves realizing that you overeat when you are bored, lonely, or stressed. One of the most nurturing gifts you can give yourself is something to help replace those feelings—and prevent you from sabotaging your eating plan. If you are lonely, join a support group or club. If you are bored, try a new hobby. If you are stressed, take a day off or treat yourself to a yoga class. Or talk to a friend—sometimes this can be an immediate form of self-care that will get you through a challenging moment.

PRACTICE AFFIRMATIONS AND VISUALIZATIONS

Try using affirmations daily as positive reinforcement for your new wellness lifestyle. Say your affirmations to yourself every morning and write them down and display them somewhere visible in your home or at your office: on a mirror, in a picture frame, on the refrigerator, on your eyeglass case, or in your wallet. You can buy pre-made affirmation cards or refer to books with positive sayings.

Positive reinforcement can also take the form of visualizations based on thoughts and memories. Remember how great you felt when you succeeded at riding a two-wheeler, operating a computer, or putting together a stereo system? Then remember how wonderful your Active Wellness efforts felt when you completed your first day of exercise or cleaned out your cupboards of unhealthy foods. Those were big accomplishments! Remembering how it feels to accomplish something worthwhile—and picturing it in your mind—brings you closer to achieving your next goal.

Sometimes, remembering even negative "achievements" can help you stay on track. Occasionally recalling how bad you felt to be out of shape, eat in unhealthy ways, or feel acutely stressed can help you stay on the wellness path—just to avoid feeling that bad again! Then use visualization to help you create an image of how it looks and feels to be successful and to achieve your goals.

DO A REALISTIC SELF-APPRAISAL

Honest self-appraisal is critical to maintaining your wellness progress. How did you see yourself at the start of your Active Wellness journey? Who are

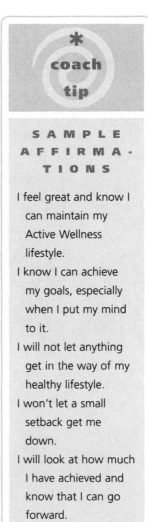

* coach tip

SAMPLE AFFIRMATIONS

I feel great and know I can maintain my Active Wellness lifestyle.

I know I can achieve my goals, especially when I put my mind to it.

I will not let anything get in the way of my healthy lifestyle.

I won't let a small setback get me down.

I will look at how much I have achieved and know that I can go forward.

you today? How capable are you of staying on course and achieving your long-term health goals?

Achieving your long-term goals takes time and patience. In order to move forward, you need to accept how far you have come. Think of your gains, no matter how small, as real progress. All your efforts may not be visible, but every change you made took effort. And every effort you've made is worth recognizing, rewarding, and positively reinforcing.

Progress is always a slow and deliberate learning process. With each step, you build upon the success you achieved in an earlier step. Step by step, you begin to weave together the fabric of a lifetime of healthy living. Without the first, small steps, followed by the slow, steady progress, your changes would never be permanent.

One helpful tool for positively reinforcing your small and large successes is to do a daily realistic appraisal of how your day went. At the end of each day, break down your experiences into several categories:

Things you or others did that pleased you
Things you wish you'd done
Things you didn't want to do but did anyway
Things you can't change

THINGS YOU OR OTHERS DID THAT PLEASED YOU Reflect on positive experiences and favorable compliments that occurred throughout your day. Cherish them. Unfortunately, we tend to accentuate the negative and forget the positive. Don't let a positive experience go by without acknowledging it and holding on to it. If someone gives you a compliment, accept it and let it make you feel good. You deserve it. When you do something that you are proud of, give yourself a pat on the back or a nurturing reward.

THINGS YOU WISH YOU'D DONE Learn from your mistakes and then move on. Nobody is perfect. When you've done something you wish you hadn't, think about how you might do things differently in the future. Mistakes are an integral part of learning. They provide essential feedback when we are learning new behaviors and tasks, which make them, ironically, vital to our going forward to eventual success. Many times, a mistake means that we're finally learning how to do something new.

THINGS YOU DIDN'T WANT TO DO BUT DID ANYWAY Sometimes we just can't help ourselves. No matter how much we know better, we still go ahead and do or say something that is counterproductive to our good health and well-being. Our stronger desires and passions get the best of us, and we yield to temptation—opting, for example, for a hot-fudge sundae instead of fresh fruit for dessert. Let those kinds of occasional slips go, forgive yourself, and move on. You're not a bad person who has no willpower. You're simply human and yielded to a little temptation. Instead of beating yourself up about occasional slips and missteps, use these situations to expand your awareness about yourself regarding your true needs and wants around a particular temptation or old pattern, whether it's eating rich desserts, neglecting exercise, or slipping back into unhealthy behaviors. Expanding your awareness helps you understand why you slipped to begin with and gives you the confidence to move forward with a greater understanding of yourself and your behaviors.

THINGS YOU CAN'T CHANGE Obsessing about things that have already happened or been said and that simply cannot be changed is a waste of time and energy. They are out of your control, so one of the best things you can do for yourself is just let them go. A useful way to let go of such experiences is to write them down and then destroy or discard them—in effect, eliminating them.

SET REALISTIC GOALS Were your original goals reasonable and realistic? Often we sabotage our chances for success when we set unrealistic goals or have grandiose expectations. We inadvertently set ourselves up to fail, then channel the energy we could have used to succeed into unhealthy behaviors or unproductive activities.

In the spaces on page 210, write down one of the short- or long-term goals that you set for yourself in Step 1 of your Active Wellness Program. Then write down the steps you took to achieve that goal. Stop at the point where you are right now with that goal and pay particular attention to the problems that you overcame and the obstacles that are still in the way of your success.

My original goal:

_____

_____

_____

_____

_____

Steps I've taken to achieve my goal:

1. _____

2. _____

3. _____

4. _____

5. _____

What else do you need to do to achieve your original goals or to reach any new goals you set for yourself? In fact, use what you learned in this assessment to establish a new, realistic short-term goal.

The best way to succeed in your Active Wellness Program is to continue to set achievable short-term goals each week, all designed to help you attain a long-term wellness goal. As you complete one goal, set a new one.

As you tackle each new short-term goal, you will encounter obstacles—new and old—along the path to success. Use your new behavior management skills to short-circuit these obstacles. If you are having real trouble achieving your short- or long-term goals, seek help from professionals and friends.

Eventually—and perhaps now—you'll be ready to set a new long-term goal for yourself. If you've been concentrating on eating well and exercising, you may want to move on to stress management. When you're ready, take a moment to record your new long-term goal and the new steps—short-term, weekly goals—that you will take to achieve that goal:

My new or current goal:

_____

_____

_____

_____

_____

I have been on the Active Wellness Program for two years now. I chose to start the program because my blood pressure was dangerously high, and I was scared. I wanted to learn how to control my blood pressure without medication. To do that, I knew I needed to learn how to lose weight and control my stress levels. Active Wellness gave me the opportunity to do both because it addressed my whole life, not just what I was eating.

I began the program by creating a healthy eating plan for myself and tracking my food portions. I really liked tracking my portions because it helped emphasize all the choices I had. Having done many diets, I was thrilled not to feel limited in my selection of foods. I soon had a great time experimenting with new foods and finding satisfying recipes to prepare. When I went shopping, it sometimes felt like a treasure hunt—I was always looking for new foods to try. I discovered new foods and had a great time! For someone who loves food, I was pleasantly surprised at how much I could enjoy eating healthy foods that would also help me take care of myself.

By the end of the first year of Active Wellness, and in time for my sixtieth birthday, I had set goals that helped me establish a regular exercise and yoga routine. My blood pressure was at low normal and I was feeling great! The positive outlook I had about taking care of myself translated to my work. I was benefiting in numerous ways, and so were my husband and family, because now that I was watching my diet more closely, so were they.

Off and on throughout the next year on the program, I found that I could slip into my old habits. But now, instead of feeling like the whole program is over, Active Wellness has taught me that I can pick myself back up again and stay focused on my health goals, and I am right back on track. I have learned that being good to myself means slowing down, thinking about what I want, and doing what it takes to get that.

This program has helped me feel great! I feel healthy, strong, and very capable of managing my stress. I am so thankful that I have had the opportunity to live the Active Wellness way. It feels so good that I don't ever plan to go back to my old way of being.

Fran, age sixty-one, dress size decreased by 2, blood pressure reduced to low normal

Steps I will take to achieve that goal:

1. _____
2. _____
3. _____
4. _____
5. _____

To celebrate your progress along the Active Wellness journey, remember the word *reward*. It will remind you to acknowledge all your gains, small and large, and to remain committed to your program. **REWARD = Recognize Every Win and Remain Driven**

BE COMPASSIONATE WITH YOURSELF

One of the best things you can do for yourself is to treat yourself with compassion. Compassion for yourself means to accept yourself. When you accept yourself, you'll find it easier to let go of the occasional relapse and get back on a healthy track. With compassion, you won't feel like a failure when you fall off the wellness path; you will simply feel human, get up, dust yourself off, and start all over again.

Compassion is equal parts understanding, acceptance, and forgiveness. With understanding, you seek to observe and learn about yourself with curiosity instead of criticism. With acceptance, you not only accept yourself and your strengths and weaknesses, but you respect others as well. You are who you are, and they are who they are. If you want to improve yourself by becoming stronger or leaner or healthier, that's great. However, the greatest strides in good health and well-being may finally occur only when you accept yourself as you are, at any time, in any moment. Then you will find yourself centered and truly at peace, and you can let go of mistakes with forgiveness.

Forgiveness means learning from the past and moving on with no regrets. Forgiveness also means that you stay rooted in the present and look forward to the future with a clean slate. Learning to sincerely forgive—yourself and others—may take time but is essential to good health and body/mind/spirit wellness. The opposite side of forgiveness is resentment, one of the most destructive feelings, which can eat away at your inner strength and sabotage the best of intentions. Forgiveness is liberation from resentment, and that liberation is nothing less than a dose of optimal good feeling.

SEEK OUT SUPPORT AND COOPERATION

Going through major changes can be very difficult, all the more so if you are doing it alone. When you have friends and family rooting for you on the sidelines, people who are genuinely concerned about your well-being, then making the hard changes somehow feels easier and less frightening.

Accepting support and encouragement from others is one of the best ways to help yourself stay committed to your goals. While the real positive reinforcement—the kind that will enable you to stick to your guns—has to come from inside you, outside support can help you get through the tough times, when you find yourself doubting your ability to continue on the Active Wellness path.

The key to finding this sort of support is effective communication—reaching out to the people in your life from whom you feel you can get support, and expressing your needs in a direct, clear manner. Of course, no one but you can take on the challenges of your Active Wellness Program, but by taking responsibility for your wellness in specific situations, such as explaining to family members or friends why you need a modified version of what is being served for dinner, and being honest with them about the things you find both rewarding and anxiety provoking in your journey, you will not only create a network of understanding and support for yourself, but you may also inspire others around you to make changes toward an Active Wellness lifestyle.

If you feel that you don't have friends and loved ones with whom you can confide, consider joining a structured support group. There are therapy and self-help-oriented groups that focus on both specific and general issues surrounding health and well-being, including breast cancer, heart disease, diabetes, and overeating problems, and where members can support each other through the sharing of their experiences.

You also can seek out a non-therapeutic type of support group, one that directly helps you actualize your Active Wellness lifestyle. This might include fitness groups that walk, jog, or cycle together. You also can join an Active Wellness Program near your home for support in making Active Wellness a lifetime goal.

USE STRATEGIES FOR MAINTAINING SUCCESS

Nobody is perfect. We all have times when maintaining our Active Wellness Program becomes difficult. Since learning new skills takes time, energy, and practice, don't be surprised if you occasionally lapse into old, unhealthy habits. Relapses are more likely to occur in high-stress situations that involve arguments, job stress, social pressure, and negative emotional states. Here are some strategies that other Active Wellness clients have successfully used when they felt they were veering off the path of wellness.

* Take things one day at a time. Just because you had trouble today doesn't mean you'll have trouble tomorrow.
* Use your new habits as substitutes for your old behaviors.
* Distract yourself with something else. Try deep breathing, smelling a nice scent, meditating on a beautiful scene, writing a letter to a friend, listening to music, taking a walk, writing down new affirmations, or reading a book.
* Work through your Active Wellness Program by trying to accomplish one realistic, short-term goal each week. Stick with the same goal until you achieve it, then move on.
* Reward yourself for your positive efforts.
* Forgive yourself for your lapses. Relapses happen to everybody. Don't beat yourself up over them. Just regain control and move on.

coach tip

PEACE: On your Active Wellness journey, if you find yourself heading down a crooked path that feels like an old habit or pattern, try your best to stop what you are doing at that moment and change your direction. The word *PEACE* can help you think through the steps to choosing a new, healthier route rather than relapsing into old behaviors.

P = Pause and take a few deep breaths
E = Experience the moment
A = Acknowledge your thoughts and feelings
C = Choose what you feel is best for you to do
E = Enjoy the choice

* Treat yourself with love and understanding. You deserve it.
* Give yourself time to notice visible results. Let longer intervals go by— two weeks or a month—before you measure yourself, weigh yourself, or do a self-appraisal.

PRIORITIZE YOUR LONG-TERM GOALS

To maintain your Active Wellness successes for a lifetime, you must learn to prioritize your long-term goals. Set your sights high, but be realistic. Make sure each new goal is reasonable, achievable, and builds on a previous goal that you've successfully accomplished. The following will help you prioritize your long-term goals for the future and assess where you are now. As you accumulate skills and knowledge, your learning speed will increase and you should find it easier to make small changes. Remember: You are in control. How far you travel in the Active Wellness Program is determined by what you choose for yourself and how you go about getting it. If you want to, you can do it.

Long-term Goals Priority List

The long-term goal(s) I have accomplished:

_____

_____

_____

_____

The long-term goal(s) I am working toward now:

_____

_____

_____

_____

The long-term goal(s) I plan to work toward in coming months/future years:

_____

_____

_____

_____

All the strategies listed in Step 7 are meant as suggestions and guides. If you have alternative solutions for helping yourself continue the Active Wellness journey, please feel free to use them. What's important is that you help yourself continue to take the road to healthy self-empowerment and a lifetime of wellness.

Main Points to Maintaining Active Wellness for a Lifetime

- ✔ Notice the changes you have made since you began reading this book and practicing Active Wellness. These are your first achievements of Active Wellness.
- ✔ In order to move along with your goals and continue to achieve on your program, recognize your success and create new goals.
- ✔ Seek out support and cooperation from close friends and family. Support can help you stay on track and committed to your goals.
- ✔ Make sure your goals and expectations are realistic, and enjoy your successes!

Congratulations! You have completed the seven steps of Active Wellness. Wherever you are in your program, that is the place you are meant to be. If you have just completed the book and plan to go back and begin the program, feel free to begin at Step 1 or start with the step that best addresses your present goals. So, if you are really ready to start exercising and that is your primary goal, you may want to begin with Step 4 instead of Step 2. If you put attention to your goal each day and focus on recording your achievements in your diary, you will move along the Active Wellness path at the rate that best works for you. Active Wellness is about creating a total lifestyle approach, so I encourage you not to stop when you have succeeded at one discipline; nutrition, exercise, stress management, and habit change. To truly feel your best each day, you will want to integrate all the disciplines together. It takes most people close to a year to really feel that they have every aspect of the program under their belt. So, enjoy your journey, take one step at a time, and you will succeed!

If you have questions or would like more information about the Active Wellness Program, go to the Web site at www.activewellness.com.

Testimonial

My weight had always been an issue, from the time of my early childhood through my adult years. At times along the way I have been in control, but for the most part I have lived my life as an obese person with elevated blood pressure. My obstacles were a lifetime of bad habits and excuses, a sedentary lifestyle, and a lack of energy. The paralyzing effects of this problem on one's self-esteem is debilitating and in my case overpowered my entire mindset. My ability to consume vast amounts of food and my weight problem permeated my every waking moment, limiting my enjoyment of life and making simple things monumental problems.

With Active Wellness, I was able to focus on a holistic approach for overall physical health through mindset as well as diet. I became aware of just how much food I was consuming—I was shocked. By setting realistic goals, tracking my food, taking vitamins, and integrating exercise into my daily routine, I was able to take control of my health and my weight. I learned how I could continue to eat some of my favorite foods, with a new health-conscious approach. With Active Wellness, I learned how to take control of my health and make informed decisions about my state of being. Using the tools and information I learned from Active Wellness, I have shed 150 pounds. I have a new lease on life, and I continue to use what I have learned.

Ed, age thirty-nine, lost 150 pounds, improved health and self-esteem

Special Dietary Guidelines

Athlete

If you are an athlete who exercises only at high intensity five to seven times per week, then you will need to add back some of the calories you expend to make sure you are getting enough fuel for your body. Use the following equation to estimate you caloric expenditure:

Caloric expenditure determined from the
Daily Calorie Intake Chart × 1.4 = _____ total calories

As an athlete, you will use your calories more efficiently over time. So, the amount you need to eat should not match the amount of energy or calories you expend, it can be less. As an athlete, make sure you are well hydrated. Take in at least two glasses of water during your training. You can use sports drinks, but be aware of the caloric intake in the drink.

Pregnant or Breast-Feeding

You will need to consume 300 more calories per day. When you are pregnant, it is helpful to take these extra calories in the form of dairy. Two extra Dairy servings will help you get the adequate increase in calories and the increase in calcium. Pregnancy also requires an increase in other nutrients such as folate, which you should have in your prenatal vitamin. Do not try to lose weight while you are pregnant, but if you are breast-feeding you can follow the weight-loss recommendations from Step 3. Avoid alcohol and caffeine if pregnant or breast-feeding.

$$\frac{\text{Total}}{\text{calories}} = \frac{\text{calorie level}}{\text{from DCIC for M}} + 300 \text{ calories}$$

Specialized Meal Plans

ACTIVE WELLNESS EATING PLAN FOR OSTEOPOROSIS PREVENTION AND MENOPAUSE

GENERAL NUTRITION GUIDELINES The United States has one of the highest rates of osteoporosis in the world. Between 15 and 20 million Americans have osteoporosis, a disease characterized by a decrease in bone mass and bone density.

This plan is based on a breakdown in energy nutrients of 50 percent carbohydrates, 25 percent proteins, and 25 percent fats. This plan emphasizes servings of high-calcium foods to meet elevated demands for those who are concerned with consuming adequate amounts of calcium to maintain bone mass and bone density. Combine this plan with the Active Wellness Basic Food and Nutrition Guidelines for a well-balanced plan that will help prevent osteoporosis and promote optimum health.

After the body reaches the age of thirty, the majority of bone is formed. From that point on, if calcium levels drop in the blood, your body extracts the calcium it needs from your bones. This depletes bone density and mass, particularly after menopause, and significantly increases the risk for serious

Active Wellness Eating Plan for Osteoporosis Prevention and Menopause

Calorie Level	Grains/ Starches	Veggie	Protein	Fruit	Dairy	Fat	Sweets	Alcohol
1,200	3	3+	3	2	3	4	1	1
1,300	4	3+	4	2	3	5	1	1
1,400	4	4+	4	2	3	5	1	1
1,500	4	4+	4	3	3	5	1	1
1,600	4	4+	5	3	3	5	1	1
1,700	5	4+	5	3	4	6	1	1
1,800	5	4+	6	3	4	6	1	1
1,900	6	4+	6	3	4	6	1	1
2,000	6	5+	7	4	4	6	1	1
2,100	7	5+	7	4	4	7	1	1
2,200	7	5+	8	4	4	8	1	1
2,300	8	5+	8	4	4	9	1	1
2,400	8	5+	8	5	4	9	1	1
2,500	9	5+	9	5	5	9	1	1
2,600	10	6+	9	5	5	10	1	1

For all calorie levels, drink a minimum of 8 glasses of water a day.

bone fractures. Therefore, you need to consume optimal levels of calcium every day, via foods and supplements, to maintain an adequate calcium balance in your body. You need to do four things to maximize calcium levels in your blood. First, take in enough calcium to meet your daily needs. Calcium is best absorbed from the foods you eat. Intake goals, based on the National Institutes of Health's consensus panel recommendations for calcium are as follows: Adolescents should consume 1,200 to 1,500 mg per day, twenty-five- to fifty-year-old adults should consume 1,000 mg per day, and females over fifty-one (or on estrogen replacement) and men over sixty-five should consume 1,500 mg per day. If you cannot meet your needs with the foods you eat (see the Calcium-Rich Foods chart on page 117), a supplement is recommended. However, do not take a calcium supplement with 2,500 mg (or more) per day, because it can raise the risk of kidney stones and interfere with the absorption of other essential minerals, such as iron, zinc, and magnesium.

Second, consume ample quantities of foods or vitamin and mineral supplements that enhance the absorption of calcium, including soy-based foods, vitamin D, and vitamin C. Soy-based foods contain phytoestrogens, which may inhibit the loss of calcium from your bones. Vitamin D is essential for the absorption and utilization of calcium. It is a nutrient naturally made by our bodies upon exposure to ten to fifteen minutes of sunlight; however, this ability declines with age. If you do not spend time outdoors or are over fifty years of age, you should consider taking a daily vitamin D supplement of 400 to 800 IU, which can be part of your calcium supplement. One cup of low-fat or skim milk is fortified with approximately 100 IU of vitamin D. Vitamin C also helps enhance the absorption of calcium. The amounts of vitamin C in the Active Wellness Eating Plans will adequately meet your requirement, but it is also a good idea to eat calcium-rich foods (yogurt, cottage cheese, milk) with fruits or vegetables that are high in vitamin C. (See the list of fruits and vegetables in the Foods Rich in Antioxidants and Other Vitamins chart in Step 4.)

Third, avoid foods and minerals that inhibit the absorption of calcium, including excess protein, salt, iron, beet greens, and spinach. Beet greens and spinach are high in calcium but are also high in substances called oxalates, which inhibit calcium absorption. Substitute soy-based food products (soybean milk, tofu, and soybeans) for some of the protein in your diet. And limit salt intake to 2,300 mg (1 teaspoon) or less per day.

Fourth, weight-bearing exercises are important to maintaining bone mass. Choose an exercise that you enjoy and try to do it for at least thirty minutes each day. If you do take calcium supplements, for best absorption, take them with food in 500 mg dosages or less, spaced throughout the day. According to recent research from Tuft University's Human Nutrition Research Center on Aging, if you are taking 1,500 mg of calcium daily you should complement this with 10 mg of zinc, because high levels of calcium inhibit zinc absorption. Check your multivitamin levels of zinc before you take an additional supplement. Another mineral that contributes to the formation of strong bones is magnesium. Magnesium is found in whole grains, nuts, beans, tofu, and dark green leafy vegetables. Your multivitamin will help ensure that you are taking in adequate levels of magnesium each day.

CAUTION: TOO MUCH OF A GOOD THING Please be aware that the National Academy of Sciences has set tolerable upper intake levels (UL) for calcium at 2,500 mg per day and vitamin D at 2,000 IU (50 mcg) per day. Health problems can occur when your daily intake is at the UL levels or above.

ACTIVE WELLNESS EATING PLAN FOR HEART DISEASE, STROKE, ELEVATED CHOLESTEROL, AND HIGH BLOOD PRESSURE

GENERAL NUTRITION GUIDELINES This plan is based on a breakdown in nutrients of 55 percent carbohydrates, 25 percent proteins, and 20 percent fats. This plan includes 5 percent more carbohydrates and 5 percent less

Active Wellness Eating Plan for Prevention of Heart Disease, Stroke, Elevated Cholesterol, and High Blood Pressure

Calorie Level	Grains/ Starches	Veggie	Protein	Fruit	Dairy	Fat	Sweets	Alcohol
1,200	3	4+	4	3	2	3	1	1
1,300	4	5+	4	3	2	3	1	1
1,400	5	5+	5	3	2	3	1	1
1,500	5	4+	5	3	2	3	1	1
1,600	5	5+	6	3	3	4	1	1
1,700	6	5+	6	3	3	4	1	1
1,800	7	5+	6	4	3	4	1	1
1,900	8	6+	6	4	3	4	1	1
2,000	8	6+	7	4	3	5	1	1
2,100	8	6+	8	5	3	5	1	1
2,200	9	6+	9	5	3	5	1	1
2,300	10	6+	9	5	3	5	1	1
2,400	10	6+	9	6	3	6	1	1
2,500	11	6+	10	6	3	6	1	1
2,600	12	6+	10	6	3	6	1	1

For all calorie levels, drink a minimum of 8 glasses of water a day.

fats than the Active Wellness Basic Eating Plan in order to help prevent diet risks associated with heart disease.

In conjunction with the general Active Wellness guidelines, which are beneficial for preventing heart disease, this plan also emphasizes potassium-rich foods and foods rich in vitamins B_6 and B_{12} and folate. Other risk factors associated with heart disease include smoking, sedentary lifestyle, and obesity.

PREVENTING HEART DISEASE, STROKE, AND ELEVATED CHOLESTEROL Reducing your risks for heart disease and stroke and lowering your cholesterol levels require that you watch your total intake of fat, trans-fatty acids, and saturated fat. Fats and elevated cholesterol can clog arteries, decreasing blood flow to the heart, causing heart disease and possible heart attacks. You can refer to the guidelines in Step 1 to reassess your risk based on your current cholesterol levels.

Aim to keep your triglyceride level below 100, since recent research from the University of Maryland's Center for Preventive Cardiology links readings above 100 with more than twice the risk for heart disease. Triglycerides can be elevated by refined sugars, processed flours, bread products, sweets, alcohol, and fat, so try to avoid these foods.

A number of recent cardiovascular research studies around the world indicate that a fourth substance in the blood, an amino acid called homocysteine, significantly increases the risk for heart attack when found in high levels. Elevated levels occur when homocysteine is not broken down properly in the body, due to a genetic or environmental defect. Recent research found that brewed coffee can elevate homocysteine and has a particularly strong effect when taken after meals—so try to eliminate this from your diet. Vitamins B_6 and B_{12} together with folate can break down homocysteine to safe levels, which is why this plan specifically recommends them. Foods rich in vitamins B_6 and B_{12} include poultry, fish, pork, beans, whole grains, fortified soy foods, lean meats, and milk. Folate can be found in leafy vegetables, legumes, and fortified cereals. It is a good idea to take the recommended folate supplement listed in the guidelines. Also check your multivitamin to see if it has at least 4 mg of vitamin B_6 and 8 mcgs of vitamin B_{12}; otherwise, feel free to add a B-complex vitamin.

Omega-3 essential fatty acids can help lower cholesterol and reduce the risk for heart disease, as discussed in the Active Wellness Basic Food and Nutrition Guidelines. The flax meal recommended daily will give you 1.8 grams of omega-3 fats. Omega-3 fats are healthy to add to your diet in an effort to prevent heart disease if you are not consuming three or more servings of omega-3 rich fish weekly. Since you will be taking the flax meal, you don't need to increase your intake of fish oils unless your triglycerides are elevated, in which case the American Heart Association recommends 2 to 4 grams of omega-3 fats. You can add omega-3 to your diet by taking a fish-oil supplement that is high in omega-3; add a 1-gram capsule daily. Be aware that a fishy odor or breath may result from taking these capsules. Also, although omega-3 supplements and vitamin E can help you, the wrong dosage may increase your risk for stroke. Therefore, be sure to consult your physician before taking fish-oil or vitamin E supplements.

It is also beneficial to consider moving toward a more vegetarian diet, because plant foods like beans are naturally low in fat, high in protective antioxidants and phytochemicals, and higher in fiber—all of which can help you reduce your risk for heart disease.

Elevated trigylcerides and low HDL and elevated blood pressure—called Syndrome X in medical circles—can be a precursor for diabetes. Therefore, be sure to read the diabetes section under the eating plans.

PREVENTING HIGH BLOOD PRESSURE High blood pressure is defined as anything at or above 140/90 ml of mercury. An optimal blood pressure is equal to or less than 120/80 ml of mercury. High blood pressure may be the result of several factors: excess weight, lack of exercise, excessive sodium intake (if you are salt sensitive), excessive fat consumption, lack of fruits and vegetables in your diet, smoking, or high levels of stress.

Too much salt in the diet is commonly believed to be a major cause of high blood pressure associated with heart disease, but in fact only half the people who have elevated blood pressure are sensitive to salt. A physician can determine if you are salt sensitive by running a test to see if you have low levels of the enzyme renin, which helps regulate blood pressure. If your renin levels are low, you are probably salt sensitive and should reduce your intake of salt (sodium) to 1 teaspoon a day or less.

However, salt intake does appear related to stroke risk. Keeping your blood pressure at normal levels is particularly important for preventing strokes. In a project conducted by the National Institutes of Health, both men and women aged sixty to eighty who reduced their excess weight and sodium intake were 50 percent more likely to maintain normal blood pressure levels without medication.

Recent research from Johns Hopkins University indicates that the mineral potassium plays a significant role in regulating blood pressure. Supplementing your diet with 2,300 mg of potassium can significantly lower blood pressure if you also get at least 2,500 mg of potassium in your food daily. While many people do take potassium in supplemental tablet form, getting your potassium through foods is the optimal way to reduce your blood pressure. The chart below lists the most potassium-rich foods by serving size. Try to incorporate as many of these foods as possible into your eating plan.

Potassium-Rich Foods		
Food	**Serving**	**Potassium (mg)**
Banana	1 large	451
Cantaloupe	1 cup	494
Dried prunes	5	313
Figs	5	666
Kidney beans	½ cup	357
Potatoes	1 large	844
Raisins	¼ cup	563
Spinach	½ cup	419
Swiss chard	½ cup	483

ACTIVE WELLNESS EATING PLAN FOR TYPE 1 INSULIN-DEPENDENT AND TYPE 2 NON-INSULIN DEPENDENT DIABETES, INSULIN RESISTANCE, CARBOHYDRATE CRAVINGS, AND HYPOGLYCEMIA

The eating plan for insulin-dependent and non-insulin dependent diabetes is designed to keep blood-sugar levels down and also reduce triglyceride and cholesterol levels. Research from Stanford University and current research from Harvard School of Public Health indicate that diabetics can reduce

Active Wellness Eating Plan for Type 1 Insulin-Dependent and Type 2 Non-Insulin Dependent Diabetes, Insulin Resistance, Carbohydrate Cravers, and Hypoglycemia*

Calorie level	Grains/ Starches	Veggie	Protein	Fruit	Dairy	Fat	Sweets	Alcohol
1,200	3	3+	4	2	2	5	1	1
1,300	3	3+	4	2	3	5	1	1
1,400	3	4+	5	3	3	5	1	1
1,500	4	4+	6	2	3	5	1	1
1,600	5	4+	6	3	3	6	1	1
1,700	5	4+	6	3	3	7	1	1
1,800	6	3+	7	3	3	7	1	1
1,900	6	3+	8	3	3	7	1	1
2,000	7	5+	8	3	4	7	1	1
2,100	7	5+	8	3	4	8	1	1
2,200	8	6+	9	4	4	8	1	1
2,300	8	6+	9	4	4	9	1	1
2,400	9	5+	10	4	4	9	1	1
2,500	11	6+	10	4	4	10	1	1
2,600	11	6+	11	5	4	10	1	1

*Sweets should be low in sugar or low in carbohydrates.

their blood-sugar levels and triglycerides by eating a diet that is slightly higher in monounsaturated fats. Therefore, this eating plan is comprised of 50 percent carbohydrates, 20 percent proteins, and 30 percent fats. This eating plan applies to those with diabetes or any of the other conditions: insulin resistance, carbohydrate cravers, and hypoglycemia—all of whom need to watch their sugars and carbohydrate in their diet.

In general, the key to keeping your body-sugar levels under control is to use food to your advantage by carefully planning mealtimes and food portions. Three main components of every meal affect the elevation of blood sugar: the type of food you eat; the amount of food you eat; and the amount of fiber in the food you eat. What is significant is to make sure you try to marry your Grains/Starches intake and Fruit intake with either protein or plant fats when you eat. Proteins and fats do not elevate your blood sugar unless they are prepared with a sweet sauce or sugar. If you want a sweet, a reduced sugar or sugar-free sweet is best, to avoid potential spikes in sugar.

Unsaturated fats have been shown to lower triglycerides, so make sure you take in your servings of Fats in the form of plant fats and stick to consuming lean proteins, as listed in the Active Wellness Shopping List, 99 percent of the time.

CHECKING YOUR BLOOD SUGARS REGULARLY It is important to check your blood sugars regularly before eating and two hours after a meal, so that you are aware of how certain foods affect your blood sugar. Artificial sweeteners are acceptable to use. Alcohol is not recommended, but if you want to drink, limit it to your one drink a day.

TIMING OF MEALS Timing of meals both to maintain blood-sugar levels if you are a Type 2 insulin-resistant or hypoglycemic is important to avoid blood-sugar plunges. If you are an insulin-dependent diabetic, it is important to regulate your meals with your insulin shots. A good rule of thumb is to avoid eating more than three servings of Grains or starchy Vegetables at any one meal: This alleviates wide swings in your blood sugar. Desserts are best eaten following a meal. Fruit, which is high in sugar, can be eaten after a meal or as a snack with either a Protein or Fat serving.

EXERCISE When you exercise, your muscles take in blood sugar as fuel, so your levels will drop. You may want to have a piece of fruit before you exercise, to prevent a drop in blood-sugar levels after exercising. This is particularly true if your blood sugars are under control. If they are elevated, you may not need to have something to add more sugar to your system before exercising. Always check with your physician about eating before exercise.

EMERGENCIES These can arise when you feel your blood sugar dropping and you start to get sweaty, disoriented, and dizzy. Always carry a few glucose tablets with you for emergencies or make sure you can get to a glass of milk—which helps bring your sugars back in a slow and steady manner.

ACTIVE WELLNESS EATING PLAN FOR INDIVIDUALS
WITH A PERSONAL OR FAMILY HISTORY OF CANCER

The Active Wellness Basic Food and Nutritional Guidelines are consistent with recommendations for cancer prevention. This plan follows those guidelines and is composed of 50 percent carbohydrates, 25 percent proteins, and 25 percent fats. This plan enhances the general plan by recommending a higher intake of fruits and vegetables that contain protective phytochemicals and antioxidants to fight the damaging free radicals linked to cancer and other diseases. The Active Wellness eating plan is also consistent with the high fiber recommendations that help prevent breast and colon cancers.

Avoid foods that have been barbecued, smoked, or pickled, since these foods have been linked with some stomach and esophagus cancers. Also

	Active Wellness Eating Plan for Individuals with a Personal or Family History of Cancer							
Calorie Level	Grains/ Starches	Veggie	Protein	Fruit	Dairy	Fat	Sweets	Alcohol
1,200	2	6+	4	3	2	4	1	1
1,300	3	6+	5	3	2	4	1	1
1,400	4	6+	5	3	2	4	1	1
1,500	4	6+	6	3	3	4	1	1
1,600	6	6+	6	3	2	5	1	1
1,700	6	6+	6	3	2	6	1	1
1,800	7	6+	7	3	2	6	1	1
1,900	7	6+	8	3	3	6	1	1
2,000	8	6+	8	3	3	6	1	1
2,100	8	6+	8	3	3	7	1	1
2,200	9	6+	9	3	3	7	1	1
2,300	9	6+	9	3	3	8	1	1
2,400	10	6+	10	4	3	8	1	1
2,500	11	6+	10	4	3	9	1	1
2,600	11	6+	11	4	3	9	1	1

For all calorie levels, drink a minimum of 8 glasses of water a day.

avoid alcohol if you are concerned about cancer of the liver, head, or neck (including the larynx, pharynx, mouth, and esophagus). Excessive alcohol intake also weakens the immune system.

If you or someone you know is undergoing radiation or chemotherapy for cancer, bear in mind the importance of consuming enough calories to keep the body strong and help promote healing. In particular, the appetite may be reduced or the taste buds impaired while undergoing chemotherapy, so finding appetizing and tasty foods is a worthy challenge. If chewing is a problem, liquid shakes and less acidic juices made with fruit and vegetables and smoothies made with soy milk or skim milk are excellent nutritional supplements.

Digestive problems If you have any of the following digestive difficulties—hiatal hernia, irritable bowl syndrome, or ulcers—it is important to eat small meals frequently, say six to eight small meals (think of them as half meals) a day. You may also need to reduce the amount of fiber in your diet. You can do this by peeling your fruits and cooking your vegetables, except lettuce. Plus, during a flare-up, avoiding acidic foods such as citrus fruits, tomatoes (raw), wine, and vinegar can be helpful. Contacting a physician to discuss your situation is advisable. You may also want to try acidophilus daily to keep the flora of your gastrointestinal tract healthy. You can find a reliable brand at www.culturelle.com.

Lactose intolerance Avoid or eliminate dairy products. Depending on the severity of your condition, you may be able to tolerate yogurt and low-fat buttermilk. Substitutions for milk are Lactaid, soy milk, or rice milk. Soy milk is usually supplemented with more calcium than rice milk. If you have a bad condition, Lactaid milk can cause discomfort.

Gluten intolerance (celiac sprue) This is an intolerance to the protein gliadin, which is found in wheat, oats, barley, and rye. If you have this condition, substitute rice, corn, buckwheat, soy, or potato.

Gout This is a condition that can come from following a high-protein diet for too long. Foods high in purine will trigger a reaction. They include organ meats, bouillon/meat broth, meat extracts, anchovies, scallops, mussels, and mackerel. Loss of excess weight also helps relieve symptoms.

Allergies Food allergies can create a range of symptoms, including nausea, itching, vomiting, rashes, asthma, and anaphylactic shock. Some of the most common food allergies derive from peanuts, tree nuts, eggs, shellfish, and wheat. In general, if you have a reaction after eating a meal and you think it is an allergy, check with your doctor and see a dietitian.

Renal disease For detailed instructions, contact your physician and make an appointment with a dietitian. The recommendations will depend upon the severity of the disease.

Sample Eating Plans

Osteoporosis Eating Plan for Women and Men

Please note that additional servings are given for men.*

Breakfast

1 Grains/Starch	1 cup dry-flake whole-grain cereal or hot cereal, or 1 slice whole-grain toast
1 Fruit	1 cup of berries or 1 piece of fruit of your choice
1 Dairy	1 cup skim milk or 1 cup low-fat soy milk
Water Equivalent	1 to 2 cups of herbal tea or water
Other	Vitamins
Other	Sprinkle flax meal on cereal (already counted as part of plan)

Snack

Water Equivalent	1 cup of hot herbal tea
2 Fats	1 handful of nuts (about 12 large nuts, or 40 peanuts)

Lunch

1 Grains/Starch	½ cup cooked beans (e.g., chickpeas, kidney beans, black beans, lentils) or 1 cup of bean soup
1 Fat	2 tablespoons low-fat salad dressing
1 Dairy	1 ounce low-fat cheese or ½ cup cottage cheese
Vegetables (Free) Equals about 3 servings of vegetables	Large salad w/ dark green lettuce or spinach, ½ cup of other vegetables that are unlimited—can include carrots, tomatoes, plus any other vegetables you would like.
1 Sweet	½ cup low-fat or fat-free frozen yogurt
Water Equivalent	2 cups (16 ounces) herbal tea, water, or sparkling water
*Men add: 2 Grains/Starch	½ cup bean salad (if oil is added to the salad—count as a fat or ½ cup pasta salad or potato salad with fat-free or low-fat dressing, or 1 ounce popcorn or low-fat or fat-free chips; or use the two grains for whole-grain bread and make a sandwich with your protein. Use veggies on sandwich and as a side salad or soup.
1 Fat	1 tablespoon of nuts or seeds
2 Protein	2 ounces of lean protein (e.g., fish, shellfish, chicken breast, turkey breast)

Osteoporosis Eating Plan (continued)

Snack

1 Fruit	1 small apple or orange or other fruit of choice
1 Dairy	1 cup (8 ounces) low-fat or fat-free yogurt
Water Equivalent	2 cups (16 ounces) herbal tea, water, or sparkling water

Dinner

3 servings of lean protein equivalent *Men add: 1 serving to make a total of 6 servings	4 ounces lean poultry, fish, beef, pork, or 6 ounces of shell fish, or 2 cups of tofu—don't hesitate to use a sauce or marinade to add flavor.
*Men add: 1 Grains/Starch	1 cup of bean soup plus an extra serving of cooked grain (½ cup) or 2 slices of bread or 1 cup of cooked grain or a whole baked potato or sweet potato
1 Fruit	1 cup berries or other fruit
1 Vegetable	½ cup steamed broccoli
2 Vegetables	Mixed salad (2 cups raw vegetables) or 2 more cooked vegetables
2 Fats	2 tablespoons low-fat salad dressing and 1 teaspoon oil (canola or olive oil for cooking)
1 Alcohol: If you do not drink, you can trade alcohol for an extra serving of anything	1 alcoholic beverage equivalent (e.g., 5 ounces wine), or 1 serving of fruit or grain (e.g., ⅓ cantaloupe melon or add an extra ½ cup of cooked grain to your meal or 1 cup bean soup)
Water Equivalent	2 cups (16 ounces) sparkling water or herbal hot or iced tea

Heart Health Eating Plan for Women and Men

Please note that additional servings are given for men.*

Breakfast

1 Grains/Starch	1 cup dry-flake whole-grain cereal or hot cereal, or 1 slice whole-grain toast
1 Fruit	1 cup of berries or 1 piece of fruit of your choice
1 Dairy	1 cup skim milk or 1 cup low-fat soy milk
Water Equivalent	1 to 2 cups of herbal tea or water
*Men add: 1 Grains/Starch	1 cup dry-flake whole-grain cereal or hot cereal, or 1 slice whole-grain toast
Other	Vitamins
Other	Sprinkle flax meal on cereal (already counted as part of plan)

Snack

Water Equivalent	1 cup of hot herbal tea
2 Fats	1 handful of nuts (about 12 large nuts, or 40 peanuts)

Lunch

1 Grains/Starch	½ cup cooked beans (e.g., chickpeas, kidney beans, black beans, lentils) or 1 cup of bean soup
1 Fat	2 tablespoons low-fat salad dressing
Vegetables (Free) Equals about 3 servings of vegetables	Large salad w/ dark green lettuce or spinach, ½ cup of other vegetables that are unlimited—can include carrots, tomatoes, plus any other vegetables you would like
1 Sweet	½ cup low-fat or fat-free frozen yogurt
Water Equivalent	2 cups (16 ounces) herbal tea, water, or sparkling water
Men add: 2 Grains/Starch	½ cup bean salad (if oil is added to the salad—count as a Fat) or ½ cup pasta salad or potato salad with fat-free or low-fat dressing, or 1 ounce popcorn or low-fat or fat-free chips; or use the two grains for whole-grain bread and make a sandwich with your protein. Use veggies on sandwich and as a side salad or soup.
1 Fat	1 tablespoon of nuts or seeds
2 Proteins	2 ounces of lean protein (e.g., fish, shellfish, chicken breast, turkey breast)

Snack

1 Fruit	1 small apple or orange or other fruit of choice
1 Dairy	1 cup (8 ounces) low-fat or fat-free yogurt
Water Equivalent	2 cups (16 ounces) herbal tea, water, or sparkling water

Heart Health Eating Plan (continued)

Dinner

4 servings of lean protein equivalent *Men add: 1 serving to make a total of 5 servings	4 ounces lean poultry, fish, beef, pork, or 6 ounces of shellfish, or 2 cups of tofu—don't hesitate to use a sauce or marinade to add flavor.
1 Grains/Starch	1 cup any cooked grain: brown rice, whole-wheat couscous, barley, whole-wheat grain pasta
*Men add: 2 Grains/Starch	1 cup of bean soup plus an extra serving of cooked grain (½ cup) or 2 slices of bread or 1 cup of cooked grain or a whole baked potato or sweet potato
1 Vegetable	½ cup steamed broccoli
2 Vegetables	Mixed salad (2 cups raw vegetables) or 2 more cooked vegetables
1 Fat	2 tablespoons low-fat salad dressing and 1 teaspoon oil (canola or olive oil for cooking)
1 Alcohol: If you do not drink, you can trade alcohol for an extra serving of anything	1 alcoholic beverage equivalent (e.g., 5 ounces wine), or 1 serving of fruit or grain (e.g., ⅓ cantaloupe melon or add an extra ½ cup of cooked grain to your meal or 1 cup bean soup)
Water Equivalent	2 cups (16 ounces) sparkling water or herbal hot or iced tea
1 Fruit	1 cup berries or other fruit

Snack

Water Equivalent	1 cup of hot herbal tea
*Men add: 1 Fruit	1 serving of fruit of your choice—½ banana, 1 apple, or 1 handful grapes

Diabetes, Insulin Resistance Carb Cravers, and Hypoglycemia Eating Plan for Women and Men

Please note that additional servings are given for men.*

Breakfast

1 Grains/Starch	1 cup dry-flake whole-grain cereal or hot cereal, or 1 slice whole-grain toast
1 Fat	6 large nuts (cashews, almonds, walnuts)
1 Dairy	1 cup skim milk or 1 cup low-fat soy milk
Water Equivalent	1 to 2 cups of herbal tea or water
*Men add: 1 Fat	6 large nuts (cashews, almonds, walnuts)
Other	Vitamins
Other	Sprinkle flax meal on cereal (already counted as part of plan)

Snack

Water Equivalent	1 cup of hot herbal tea
2 Fats	1 handful of nuts (about 12 large nuts, or 40 peanuts)

Lunch

1 Grains/Starch	½ cup cooked beans (e.g., chickpeas, kidney beans, black beans, lentils) or 1 cup of bean soup
1 Fat	2 tablespoons low-fat salad dressing
Vegetables (Free) Equals about 3 servings of vegetables	Large salad w/ dark green lettuce or spinach, ½ cup of other vegetables that are unlimited—can include carrots, tomatoes, plus any other vegetables you would like
1 Sweet	½ cup low-fat or fat-free frozen yogurt
Water Equivalent	2 cups (16 ounces) herbal tea, water, or sparkling water
*Men add: 1 Grains/Starch	½ cup bean salad (if oil is added to the salad—count as a Fat) or ½ cup pasta salad or potato salad with fat-free or low-fat dressing, or 1 ounce popcorn or low-fat or fat-free chips; or use the two grains for whole-grain bread and make a sandwich with your protein. Use veggies on sandwich and as a side salad or soup.
1 Fat	1 tablespoon of nuts or seeds
3 Protein	3 ounces of lean protein (e.g., fish, shellfish, chicken breast, turkey breast)

Snack

1 Fruit	1 small apple or orange or other fruit of choice
1 Dairy	1 cup (8 ounces) low-fat or fat-free yogurt
1 Fat	1 serving of nuts (6 large, or 20 small)
*Men add:	an additional serving of nuts
Water Equivalent	2 cups (16 ounces) herbal tea, water, or sparkling water

Diabetes, Insulin Resistance Carb Cravers, and Hypoglycemia Eating Plan (continued)

Dinner

4 servings of lean protein equivalent *Men add: 1 serving to make a total of 5 servings	4 ounces lean poultry, fish, beef, pork, or 6 ounces of shell fish, or 2 cups of tofu—don't hesitate to use a sauce or marinade to add flavor.
1 Grains/Starch	1 cup any cooked grain: brown rice, whole-wheat couscous, barley, whole-wheat grain pasta
Men add: 1 Grains/Starch	1 cup of bean soup plus an extra serving of cooked grain (½ cup) or 2 slices of bread or 1 cup of cooked grain or a whole baked potato or sweet potato
1 Vegetable	½ cup steamed broccoli
2 Vegetables	Mixed salad (2 cups raw vegetables) or 2 more cooked vegetables
2 Fats	2 tablespoons low-fat salad dressing and 1 teaspoon oil (canola or olive oil for cooking)
1 Alcohol: If you do not drink, you can trade alcohol for an extra serving of anything	1 alcoholic beverage equivalent (e.g., 5 ounces wine), or 1 serving of fruit or grain (e.g., ⅓ cantaloupe melon or add an extra ½ cup of cooked grain to your meal or 1 cup bean soup)
Water Equivalent	2 cups (16 ounces) sparkling water or herbal hot or iced tea
*Men add: 1 Fruit	1 cup berries or other fruit

Snack

Water Equivalent	1 cup of hot herbal tea
*Men add: 1 Grain/Starch	1 serving of whole-grain crackers
1 Fat	2 teaspoons of peanut butter or other nut butter

Cancer Prevention Eating Plan for Women and Men

Please note that additional servings are given for men.*

Breakfast

1 Grains/Starch	1 cup dry-flake whole-grain cereal or hot cereal, or 1 slice whole-grain toast
1 Fruit	1 cup of berries or 1 piece of fruit of your choice
½ Dairy	½ cup skim milk or ½ cup low-fat soy milk
Water Equivalent	1 to 2 cups of herbal tea or water
*Men add: 1 Grains/Starch	1 cup dry-flake whole-grain cereal or hot cereal, or 1 slice whole-grain toast
Other	Vitamins
Other	Sprinkle flax meal on cereal (already counted as part of plan)

Snack

Water Equivalent	1 cup of hot herbal tea
2 Fats	1 handful of nuts (about 12 large nuts, or 40 peanuts)

Lunch

1 Grains/Starch	½ cup cooked beans (e.g., chickpeas, kidney beans, black beans, lentils) or 1 cup of bean soup
1 Fat	2 tablespoons low-fat salad dressing
Vegetables (Free) Equals about 3 servings of vegetables	Large salad w/ dark green lettuce or spinach, ½ cup of other vegetables that are unlimited—can include carrots, tomatoes, plus any other vegetables you would like.
1 Sweet	½ cup low-fat or fat-free frozen yogurt
Water Equivalent	2 cups (16 ounces) herbal tea, water, or sparkling water
*Men add: 2 Grains/Starch	½ cup bean salad (if oil is added to the salad—count as a Fat) or ½ cup pasta salad or potato salad with fat-free or low-fat dressing, or 1 ounce popcorn or low-fat or fat-free chips; or use the two grains for whole-grain bread and make a sandwich with your protein. Use veggies on sandwich and as a side salad or soup.
1 Fat	1 tablespoon nuts or seeds
2 Protein	2 ounces of lean protein (e.g., fish, shellfish, chicken breast, turkey breast)

Snack

1 Fruit	1 small apple or orange or other fruit of choice
1 Dairy	1 cup (8 ounces) low-fat or fat-free yogurt
Water Equivalent	2 cups (16 ounces) herbal tea, water, or sparkling water

Dinner

4 servings of lean protein equivalent *Men add: 1 serving to make a total of 5 servings	4 ounces lean poultry, fish, beef, pork, or 6 ounces of shellfish, or 2 cups of tofu—don't hesitate to use a sauce or marinade to add flavor.
*Men add: 2 Grains/Starch	1 cup of bean soup plus an extra serving of cooked grain (½ cup) or 2 slices of bread or 1 cup of cooked grain or a whole baked potato or sweet potato
1 Vegetable	½ cup steamed broccoli
2 Vegetables	Mixed salad (2 cups raw vegetables) or 2 more cooked vegetables
2 Fats	2 tablespoons low-fat salad dressing and 1 teaspoon oil (canola or olive oil for cooking)
1 Alcohol: If you do not drink, you can trade alcohol for an extra serving of anything	1 alcoholic beverage equivalent (e.g., 5 ounces wine), or 1 serving of fruit or grain (e.g., ⅓ cantaloupe melon or add an extra ½ cup of cooked grain to your meal or 1 cup bean soup)
Water Equivalent	2 cups (16 ounces) sparkling water or herbal hot or iced tea
1 Fruit	1 cup berries or other fruit

Make copies of these pages for your use.

Daily Allowance Card

	No.	☐ Daily Vitamins and Supplements		
Water				
Grains & Starches				
Veggie				
Protein				
Fruits				
Dairy				
Fats				
Sweets				
Alcohol				

Be sure to use only the number of servings allowed for your calorie level.

Goal Chart
Long-Term Goal

_____

_____

_____

_____

Short-Term Goals

_____

_____

_____

_____

Date:_____   Eating Plan Weekly Goal:_____

Daily Food Diary

Time of Day	Food Eaten	Amount	Were you hungry before you ate? Yes/No

Daily Fitness and Stress Management Diary

Time of Day	Activity	Level of Intensity	Did you meet your goal?

Personalized Exercise Program (P.E.P.) Worksheet

Current Activity Level: _____   Goal Activity Level: _____

Initial Fitness Goal: _____

Target Heart Rate Range: _____

Selected Aerobic Activities: _____

Maximum Heart Rate: _____

Days of the Week	Warm-Ups (check off the days you do aerobic activities)	Aerobic Routine		Strength-Training Routine	Stretching Routine	Cool Down/ Cool-Down Stretching (check off the days you do aerobic activities)
		Aerobic Activity	Exercise Time			
Monday						
Tuesday						
Wednesday						
Thursday						
Friday						
Saturday						
Sunday						

Bibliography

American College of Sports Medicine. *Fitness Book.* Champaign, Ill.: Leisure Press, 1992.

American College of Sports Medicine. *Resource Manual for Guidelines for Exercise Testing and Prescription,* 2nd ed. Philadelphia: William and Wilkins, 1993.

American Council on Exercise. *Personal Trainer Manual.* Boston: Reebok University Press, 1991.

Anderson, B. *Stretching.* Bolinas, Calif.: Shelter Publications, Inc., 1980.

Birkedahl, N. *The Habit Control Workbook.* Oakland, Calif.: New Harbinger Publications, Inc., 1990.

Christensen, A. *The American Yoga Association Beginner's Manual.* New York: Simon & Schuster, 1997.

Clark, N. *Sports Nutrition Guidebook.* Champaign, Ill.: Leisure Press, 1990.

Coleman, E. *Eating for Endurance,* 3rd ed. Palo Alto, Calif.: Bull Publishing Co., 1992.

Corriher, S. *Cookwise.* New York: William Morrow & Co., Inc., 1997.

Craig, S., J. Haigh, and S. Harrar. *The Complete Book of Alternative Nutrition.* Emmaus, Pa.: Rodale Press, 1997.

Dalton, S. *Overweight and Weight Management.* New York: Aspen Publishers, Inc., 1997.

Daviglus, M. L., et al. "Fish Intake and Risk of Myocardial Infarction." *New England Journal of Medicine* Vol. 336, 1997.

Dietz, W. H., and S. L. Gortmaker. "Do We Fatten Our Children at the Television Set? Obesity and Television Viewing in Children and Adolescents." *Pediatrics* Vol. 75, 1985.

Drummond, K., and J. F. Vastano. *Cook's Healthy Handbook.* New York: John Wiley & Sons, Inc., 1993.

Duerr, M. *Above and Below the Belt.* Tucson, Ariz.: Canyon Ranch Management, 1989.

Edwards, B. *America's Favorite Drug—Caffeine.* Berkeley, Calif.: Odian Press, 1992.

Environmental Nutrition: The Newsletter of Food, Nutrition, and Health. 1997–January 2003.

Erasmus, U. *Fats That Heal and Fats That Kill.* Canada: Alive Books, 1993.

Eriksson, J., et al. "Aerobic Endurance Exercise or Circuit-Type Resistance Training for Individuals with Impaired Glucose Tolerance?" *Hormone and Metabolic Research* Vol. 30, 1998.

Fescanich, D., et al. "Protein Consumption and Bone Fractures in Women." *American Journal of Epidemiology* Vol. 143, 1996.

Foreyt, J., and K. Goodrick. "The Ultimate Triumph of Obesity." *Lancet* Vol. 346, 1995.

Fragakis, Allison, S. *The Health Professional's Guide to Popular Dietary Supplements.* American Dietetic Association, 2003.

Fried, R. E., et al. "The Effect of Filtered Coffee Consumption on Plasma Lipid Levels: Results of a Randomized Clinical Trial." *JAMA* Vol. 267, 1992.

Gaede, Peter, M.D., et al. "Multifactorial Intervention and Cardiovascular Disease in Patients with Type 2 Diabetes." *New England Journal of Medicine* Vol. 348 No.5, 2003.

Groppel, J., N. Hall, and J. Loehr. *Optimal Health*. Niles, Ill.: Nightingale Conant Corporation. Audiocassette, 1996.

Harvard School of Public Health. *www.hsph.harvard.edu*. Nutrition Source. March 2003.

Health Quarterly. The Berkshire Eagle. Winter 2003.

Indiana Soybean Development Council. *Soy Facts for Dietitians,* 1996.

Jones, S. *How to Meditate*. New Canaan, Conn.: Keats Publishing, Inc., 1997.

Kabat-Zinn, J. *Full Catastrophe Living: Using the Wisdom of Your Body and Mind to Face Stress, Pain, and Illness*. New York: Delacorte Press, 1990.

Kannel, W. B., and R. C. Ellison. "Alcohol and Coronary Heart Disease: The Evidence for a Protective Effect." *Clinica Chimica Acta* Vol. 246, 1996.

Kline, D. A. *Nutrition & Immunity—Part I: Immune Components and Nutrients,* 3rd ed. Ashland, Or: Nutrition Dimension, Inc., 1995.

Kuczarmanski, R. J., et al. "Increasing Prevalence of Overweight Among U.S. Adults: The National Health and Nutrition Examination Surveys, 1960–1991." *JAMA* Vol. 272, 1994.

LaForge, R. "Mind-Body Fitness: Encouraging Prospects for Primary and Secondary Prevention." *Journal Cardiovascular Nursing,* 1997.

Lagatree, K. *Feng Shui*. New York: Villard, 1996.

Layman, Donald, Ph.D.; Richard Matts, MPH, Ph.D., R.D.; and Cathy Nonas, MS, R.D., CDE. *Emerging Health Benefits of Dietary Protein and Its Role in Weight Management*. American Dietetics Association National Conference. October 2002.

Lazarus, R., and S. Folkman. *Stress, Appraisal, and Coping*. New York: Springer Publishing Co., 1984.

Mahan, K., and M. Arlin. *Krause's Food, Nutrition, and Diet Therapy,* 8th ed. Philadelphia: W. B. Saunders and Company, 1992.

Marcus, B. H., and L. H. Forsyth. "The Challenge of Behavior Change." *Medicine and Health,* September 1997.

Margen, S. *The Wellness Nutrition Counter*. New York: Rebus, 1997.

McConnaughy, E., et al. "Stages of Change in Psychotherapy: A Follow-up Report." *Psychotherapy* Vol. 4, 1989.

Miles, E. *Tune Your Brain—Using Music to Manage Your Mind, Body, and Mood*. New York: Berkley Books, 1997.

Moore, K. A., and J. A. Blumenthal. "Exercising Training as an Alternative Treatment for Depression Among Older Adults." *Alternative Therapies in Health and Medicine* Vol. 77, 1998.

Moore, M. *How to Master Change in Your Life.* Minneapolis, Minn.: Eckankar, 1997.

NIH Consensus Development Panel. "Physical Activity and Cardiovascular Health." *JAMA* Vol. 276, 1996.

Nutrition Action Newsletter. Washington D.C., 1997.

Nutrition and the MD. "Dietary Factors Controlling Homocystine and Cardiovascular Risk." University of California, San Diego Vol. 9, 1997.

Nutrition and the MD. "Is Stored Iron a Risk for Heart Disease or Cancer?" University of California, San Diego Vol. 7, 1997.

Ornish, D. *Dr. Dean Ornish's Program for Reversing Heart Disease.* New York: Ballantine Books, 1990.

Ornstein, R., and D. Sobel. *Healthy Pleasures.* New York: Addison-Wesley, 1989.

Remen, R. *Open Your Heart Retreat.* Berkeley, Calif.: Conference Recording Services. Audiocassette, 1993.

Rock, C. L., R. A. Jacob, and P. E. Bowen. "Update on the Biological Characteristics of the Antioxidant Macronutrients: Vitamin C, Vitamin E, and Carotenoids." *Journal of the American Dietetic Association* Vol. 96, 1996.

Rossman, M. *Healing Yourself.* New York: Pocket Books, 1989.

Sapolsky, R. *Why Zebras Don't Get Ulcers.* New York: W. H. Freeman & Co., 1994.

Schwartz, B. *Diets Don't Work.* Houston, Tex.: Breakthrough Publishing, 1985.

Segar, M. L., et al. "The Effect of Aerobic Exercise on Self-Esteem and Depressive and Anxiety Symptoms Among Breast Cancer Survivors." *Oncology Nursing Forum* Vol. 25, 1998.

Seligman, M. *Learned Optimism.* New York: Simon & Schuster, 1990.

Simopoulos, A., V. Herbert, and B. Jacobson. *Genetic Nutrition.* New York: Macmillan Publishing Co., 1993.

Smith, C. Sidney, et al. "AHA/ACC Guidelines for Preventing Heart Attack and Death in Patients with Atherosclerotic Cardiovascular Disease: 2001 Update." American Heart Association: Circulation. Vol. 104, 2001.

Strecher, V. J., et al. "Goal Setting as a Strategy for Health Behavior Change." *Health Education Quarterly* Vol. 22, 1995.

Sutherland, V., and C. Cooper. *Understanding Stress: A Psychological Perspective for Health Professionals.* New York: Chapman and Hall, 1990.

Tufts University Health and Nutrition Letter. June 1996–April 1998.

UCLA Berkeley School of Public Health. *The Wellness Supermarket Shopper's Guide.* USA: Health Letter Associates, 1997.

University of CA at Berkeley, *The Wellness Encyclopedia of Food and Nutrition.* New York: Rebus, 1992.

U.S. Food and Drug Administration. Letter to Manufacturers Regarding Botanicals and Other Novel Ingredients in Conventional Foods: Center for Food Safety and Applied Nutrition: January 30, 2001.

U.S. Department of Agriculture, Human Nutrition Information Service, Leaflet No. 572, August 1992.

USDA Nutrient Database for Standard Reference, Release 13. "Nutrients in 100g of Tree Nuts." Fall 1999.

University of California Berkeley Wellness Letter. December 1996–August 1997.

Vayda, W. *Mood Foods.* Berkeley, Calif.: Ulysses Press, 1995.

Venolia, C. *Healing Environments.* Berkeley, Calif.: Celestial Arts, 1988.

Wallberg-Henriksson, H., J. Rincon, and J. R. Zierath. "Exercise in the Management of Non-Insulin Dependent Diabetes Mellitus." *Sports Medicine* Vol. 25, 1998.

Webb, D., and S. Smith. *Foods for Better Health: Prevention and Healing of Disease.* Linwood, Ill.: Publications International, Ltd., 1994.

Williams, P. T. "Relationship of Heart Disease Risk Factors to Exercise Quantity and Intensity." *Archives of Internal Medicine* Vol. 158, 1998.

Willis, J., ed. "FDA Consumer: Focus on Food Labeling." USDA: 1993.

Willis, P. *Visualization.* Chicago: NTC Publishing Group, 1994.

Winter, Metta. Pills Can't Mimic Nature's Mix of Nutrients. ALS News: Agriculture and Life Sciences. Cornell University: College of Agriculture and Life Sciences, September 2002.

Index

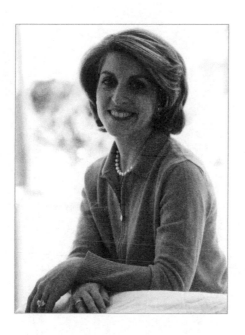

GAYLE REICHLER, M.S., R.D., CDN, is a wellness coach and dietitian. She is the founder of Active Wellness, a lifestyle and wellness program, and has helped thousands of people achieve their weight-management and health goals. She is also the creator of Gayle's Miracles (www.gaylesmiracles.com), a delicious low-calorie, low-fat chocolate truffle that is a true testimonial to her belief that healthy living should be satisfying!